Cytopathology of the Endometrium
Direct Intrauterine Sampling

ASCP Theory and Practice of Cytopathology 2

William W. Johnston, MD, Series Editor
Duke University Medical Center

Cytopathology of the Endometrium
Direct Intrauterine Sampling

Liang-Che Tao, MD, FRCPC

Professor of Pathology and Laboratory Medicine
Indiana University School of Medicine
Director, Division of Cytopathology
Indiana University Medical Center
Indianapolis, Indiana

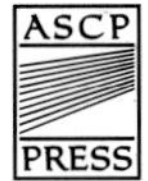

American Society of Clinical Pathologists
Chicago

Publishing Team

Jeffrey Carlson (design/production)
Shannon Hansford (marketing)
Andrea Meenahan (illustrations)
Philip Rogers (editorial)
Joshua Weikersheimer (acquisitions/development)

Notice

Library of Congress Cataloging-in-Publication Data

Tao, Liang-Che.
   Cytopathology of the endometrium: direct intrauterine sampling/Liang-Che Tao.
      p. 142
   Includes bibliographical references and index.
   ISBN 0-89189-363-6
   1. Endometrium—Cytopathology. 2. Endometrium—Cytodiagnosis. 3. Endometrium—Biopsy. I. Title.
   [DNLM: 1. Endometrium—cytology. 2. Endometrium—pathology. 3. Endometrial neoplasms—pathology. 4. Endometrial neoplasms—diagnosis. 5. Cytodiagnosis—methods. 6. Cytodiagnosis—instrumentation. WP 458 T1712c 1993]
   RG316.T36 1993
   618.1'4—dc20
   DNLM/DLC   93-4916
   for Library of Congress   CIP

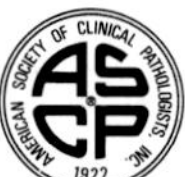

Printed in Hong Kong

97 96 95 94 93   5 4 3 2 1

To my wife, Pauline, and our children, Lorraine, Sharon, Eric, and Kevin

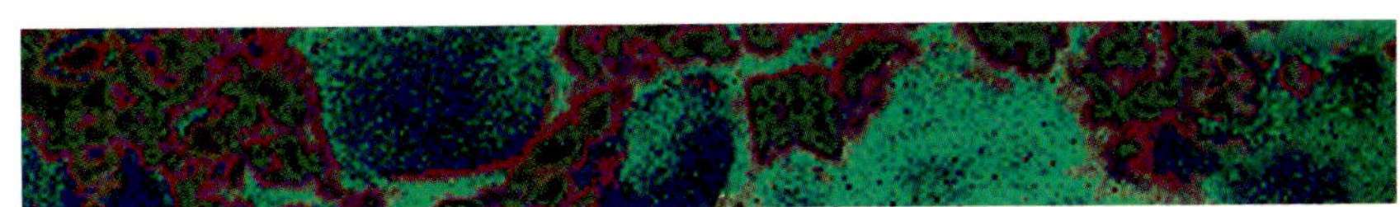

◉ Contents

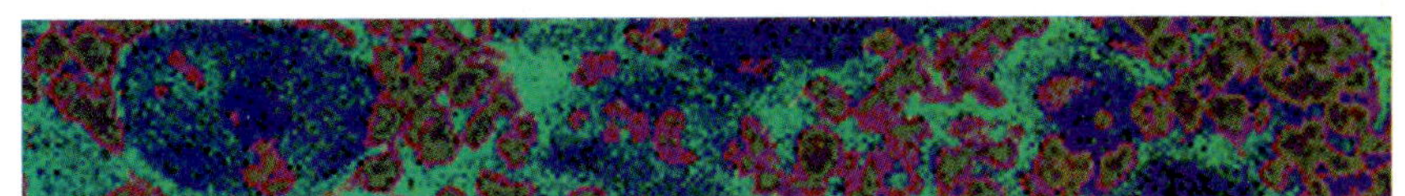

◙ Tables and Figures

◉ Preface

Endometrial carcinoma is the most common invasive neoplasm of the female reproductive tract. The incidence of endometrial carcinoma in women 45 years or older has been steadily increasing over the past few decades. There is growing need for improved early detection of endometrial carcinoma and its precursors. Case-finding procedures have generally not been used for asymptomatic women, even though many risk factors have been well documented. In addition, the duration of occult disease may be as long as 5.5 years, providing ample time for detection with an annual surveillance program.

Procedures for detection of occult uterine pathology have been studied, and efforts have been made to develop a cost-effective and reliable means of cytologic evaluation of the endometrium. A variety of devices have been developed for direct sampling of the endometrium. However, the devices previously designed for endometrial cytologic sampling do not allow reliable and consistent procurement of an adequate, representative sample (based on our experience with sampling tests using hysterectomy specimens and/or clinical trials). Published reports of endometrial cytology contain few details of specific diagnostic features to be detected for neoplastic or preneoplastic conditions. Thus, endometrial cytology has not gained wide acceptance by pathologists and gynecologists.

After reviewing over 6,000 endometrial cytologic samples obtained with various devices at the Toronto General Hospital, Toronto, Canada, over a period of 20 years, I am convinced that these obstacles can be overcome by improving the sampling device and by developing reproducible cytologic criteria for diagnosis of various pathologic and nonpathologic states in the endometrium. An improved disposable endometrial sampler (the IUMC Endometrial Sampler) has been developed at the Indiana University Medical Center. In our clinical trials and sampling tests using hysterectomy specimens, adequate, representative endometrial samples without contamination from endocervix and vagina were consistently obtained.

During the past 2 years, we procured endometrial brushing specimens by using the IUMC Endometrial Sampler prior to elective hysterectomy and/or by directly brushing resected hysterectomy specimens. The cytologic findings were correlated with histologic diagnoses, and we have used this material in addition to those histologically proven cases from my file to establish reproducible cytologic criteria for diagnosis of various pathologic and nonpathologic states in the endometrium. Both the endometrial sampling device and the specific, cytologic diagnostic criteria for the interpretation of endometrial brushing specimens are discussed and illustrated in this book.

With the help of this newly developed, improved endometrial sampling device and specific, cytologic diagnostic criteria for endometrial lesions, I hope that endometrial cytology, which was the focus of great interest in the 1970s, will be revitalized and popularized. This is a case-finding procedure and also a simple, safe office technique. I believe that family physicians should and can play an important role in screening patients for occult endometrial cancer. A previous knowledge of intrauterine device insertion is all that is required; in fact, the IUMC Endometrial Sampler has a smaller diameter and should be easier to use than the instruments employed for inserting intrauterine contraceptive devices. Let us work together to deter the rising incidence of endometrial carcinoma, especially at a time when the incidence rate is expected to increase further over the next few decades because of an expanding geriatric population.

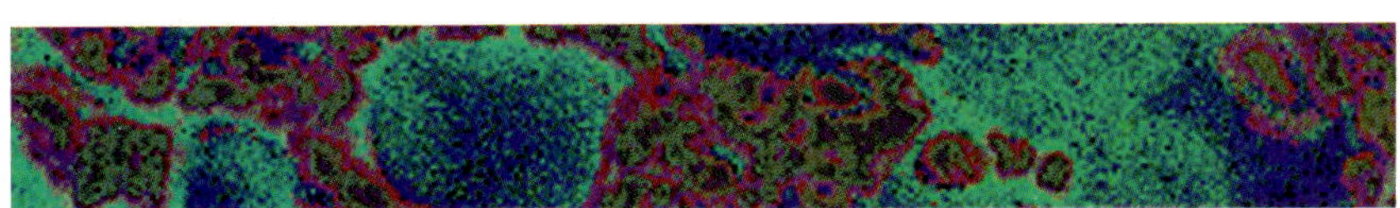

CHAPTER ONE

Direct Intrauterine Sampling in Cytology

In the last few decades, the treatment of epithelial dysplasia and carcinoma in situ of the uterine cervix detected by preventive Papanicolaou smears has significantly reduced the incidence of cervical carcinoma. Endometrial carcinoma is now the most common invasive neoplasm of the female reproductive tract, and occurs more than twice as frequently as cervical carcinoma.[6] The incidence of endometrial adenocarcinoma in women older than 45 years has been steadily increasing over the past few decades, reflecting a trend that has been reported in many countries throughout the world, including England, Canada, Norway, and Japan.[30] With an expanding geriatric population over the next few decades, the incidence rate is expected to increase further. There is a growing need for improved early detection of endometrial adenocarcinoma and its precursors. Of particular interest with respect to early detection are the "Type II" or nonestrogen-related carcinomas; these are often advanced at diagnosis, may not enlarge the uterus, and behave aggressively.[3,10]

Over 90% of new cases of endometrial carcinoma occur in women 50 years of age or older, and the majority of these are diagnosed only after the onset of symptoms related to the disease. Case-finding procedures are not regularly used for asymptomatic women, even though risk factors such as estrogen intake, obesity, diabetes, hypertension, nulliparity, ovarian tumors or polycystic ovarian disease, and late-onset menopause have all been well documented.[11,13,18,32-34] In addition, the duration of occult disease may be as long as 5.5 years,[19,20] providing ample time for early detection with an annual surveillance program. However, in the majority of cases, no test for endometrial carcinoma and its precursors, other than a Papanicolaou smear, is routinely performed. As the overall detection rate of endometrial cancer by Papanicolaou smear is unacceptably low, a more reliable test is required to provide effective case-finding for these patients.

Procedures for the detection of occult uterine pathology have been studied for many years, and numerous efforts have been made to develop a cost-effective and reliable means of cytologic evaluation of the endometrium.[1,2,4,7-9,12,14,15,23,27-29,31] A variety of devices have been developed for direct sampling of the endometrium. Some of these are commercially available. However, endometrial cytology has not gained wide acceptance by pathologists and gynecologists. There are a number of interrelated reasons for this, the most important being:

1. The devices previously designed for endometrial cytologic sampling do not allow reliable and consistent procurement of an adequate, representative sample of the entire endometrium even when properly used. This increases false-negative results. Some of them, eg, Endo-Pap (Sherwood Medical, St Louis, MO) and Mi-Mark Helix (Simpson Bayse Inc, Wilmington, DE), also have design faults that lead to inevitable contamination from endocervical and/or vaginal cells, providing sources of diagnostic errors.

2. Cytologic preparations from endometrium are more difficult to evaluate than cervicovaginal smears since many of the epithelial changes are better characterized on the squamous epithelium than on endometrial glandular cells. The criteria for cytodiagnosis of neoplastic and especially "preneoplastic" conditions of the endometrium are not as well-established as the criteria for the cytodiagnosis of cervical carcinoma and its precursors. Published reports of endometrial cytology contain few details of specific diagnostic features for neoplastic or preneoplastic conditions. Some common yet important practical problems in the interpretation of endometrial preparations, such as "the cytologic differentiation among proliferative endometrium, endometrial hyperplasia, and well-differentiated adenocarcinoma of the endometrium," to my knowledge, are not clearly discussed in the literature, and no criteria have been given for the differentiation. Therefore, a pathologist attempting endometrial cytodiagnosis for the first time may lack confidence in his or her diagnostic skill. This in turn makes the clinician attempting endometrial sampling for the first time unconvinced of its utility.

After reviewing over 6,000 endometrial cytologic samples by using various devices at the Toronto General Hospital, Toronto, Canada, over a period of 20 years, I am convinced that these obstacles can be overcome by properly designing a sampling instrument that can obtain an adequate, representative sample of the entire endometrium, and by developing reproducible, specific cytologic criteria for diagnosis of various pathologic and nonpathologic conditions in the endometrium. Both will be discussed in this book.

Basic Requirements for Endometrial Cytologic Sampling

There are three basic requirements for a good endometrial sampling

The devices previously designed for endometrial cytologic sampling do not allow reliable and consistent procurement of an adequate, representative sample of the entire endometrium

Table 1.1

General Comparison of Endometrial Sampling Devices

Brand	Diameter (mm)	Successful Insertion (%)	Adequate Sample (%)
Mi–Mark	3.5	90.4	89.4[25]
		—	90.0[5]
Endocyte	2.6	95.0	92.0[22]
Endo-Pap	2.0	90.0	89.5[25]
Isaacs	1.9	90.8	90.0[16]
		—	91.0[35]

device to detect a focal lesion and obtain a high accuracy in diagnosing neoplastic and nonneoplastic conditions:

1. Avoidance of contamination from endocervix and vagina. Contaminants from the endocervix and vagina in an endometrial sample are considered to be sources of diagnostic error. Normal endocervical cells may be mistaken for endometrial cells in the secretory phase. Reactive or atypical endocervical cells are common findings in Papanicolaou smears and may be encountered in many conditions. If these cells are present in an endometrial sample and are mistakenly interpreted as endometrial in origin, erroneous diagnoses can result. Metaplastic squamous cells of the cervical epithelium in an endometrial sample may be mistaken as squamous metaplasia of the endometrium, or as a component of adenocarcinoma (adenoacanthoma).

2. Procurement of an adequate, representative sample of the entire endometrium. Generally speaking, early pathologic lesions tend to be small and show focal changes only. If the endometrial sampling covers only part of the endometrial cavity, a significant abnormality can be missed.

3. The procedure should be safe, easy for clinical use, and well tolerated by patients. A device designed for a case-finding procedure for occult endometrial carcinoma and its precursors should be usable as a simple tool for an annual surveillance program. Therefore, the device has to be noninvasive or minimally invasive, cost-effective, and user-friendly in order to be accepted by primary care physicians and by patients for repeated tests.

In the last few decades, many cytologic devices and techniques for direct endometrial sampling have been developed. Some of the endometrial sampling devices are commercially available in the United States, including Endocyte (Gyneco Inc, Branchberg, NJ),[9,14] Endo-Pap,[8] Mi-Mark Helix,[1,14] and Isaacs Endometrial Cell Sampler (Kendall, Boston, MA).[2] The instrument diameters, success rate of insertion, and the percentage of adequate samples procured are compared in Table 1.1. The amount of pain, complications, and reported findings on the instruments' yield compared with histologic yield from dilation and curettage procedures are displayed in Table 1.2.

In our clinical trials and sampling tests using surgically resected hysterectomy specimens, none of these devices has constantly met all of the basic requirements, and we believe that there is room for further improvement. In consideration of the shortcomings present in the previ-

Table 1.2
Comparison of Acceptability, Safety, and Yield of Endometrial
Sampling Devices

Brand	Pain	Complications	Yield (%)[*]
Mi–Mark	None or mild	None	93.3 for cancer[5] 69.2 for hyperplasia[5]
Endocyte	None or mild	None	100 for cancer[9] 80.5 for hyperplasia[9]
Endo-Pap	None or mild	None	95.0 for cancer[28] 46.5 for hyperplasia[25]
Isaacs	None or mild	None	100 for cancer[2] 96.3 cumulative[35]

[*] Percent yield compared with dilation and curettage.

ously designed devices and the basic requirements for a good endometrial sampling device, an improved disposable endometrial sampler has been developed at the Indiana University Medical Center, Indianapolis, Indiana, and manufactured by Cook Ob/Gyn (Spencer, IN). Its distinguishing features are a 5-cm brush, which allows sampling of the entire endometrial cavity without excessive manipulation of the device or "scraping" of the cavity, and an 18-cm outer tube, which prevents contamination of the specimen by endocervical cells. The brush sampler has a blunt end and flexible core to prevent injury to the myometrium. The handle of the sampler has a scale enabling precise retraction of the outer tube, and the extra-long handle makes the endometrial sampling easy to maneuver for women of all body sizes, including obese patients. This new device is named the IUMC Endometrial Sampler, and with its use, the sampling technique is a simple, safe office procedure. The procedure of endometrial sampling using the IUMC Endometrial Sampler is displayed in Figure 1.1.

Advantages of Direct Endometrial Cytologic Sampling

The IUMC Endometrial Sampler is not designed to be a substitute for curettage. This device is intended for early detection of endometrial carcinoma and its precursors. For this purpose, the advantages of intra-uterine sampling using the IUMC Endometrial Sampler as compared with curettage are apparent:

1. The patient does not need general anesthesia and does not require any treatment after the procedure since there are no open wounds. This procedure can be performed in a physician's office.
2. When properly used, the endometrial sample obtained with the IUMC Endometrial Sampler contains exfoliated cells from the entire surface of the uterine cavity, whereas with an endometrial biopsy one obtains a sample from only a very small area. One might miss an endometrial carcinoma located in cornua with a regular complete curettage.

The IUMC Endometrial Sampler is intended for early detection of endometrial carcinoma and its precursors

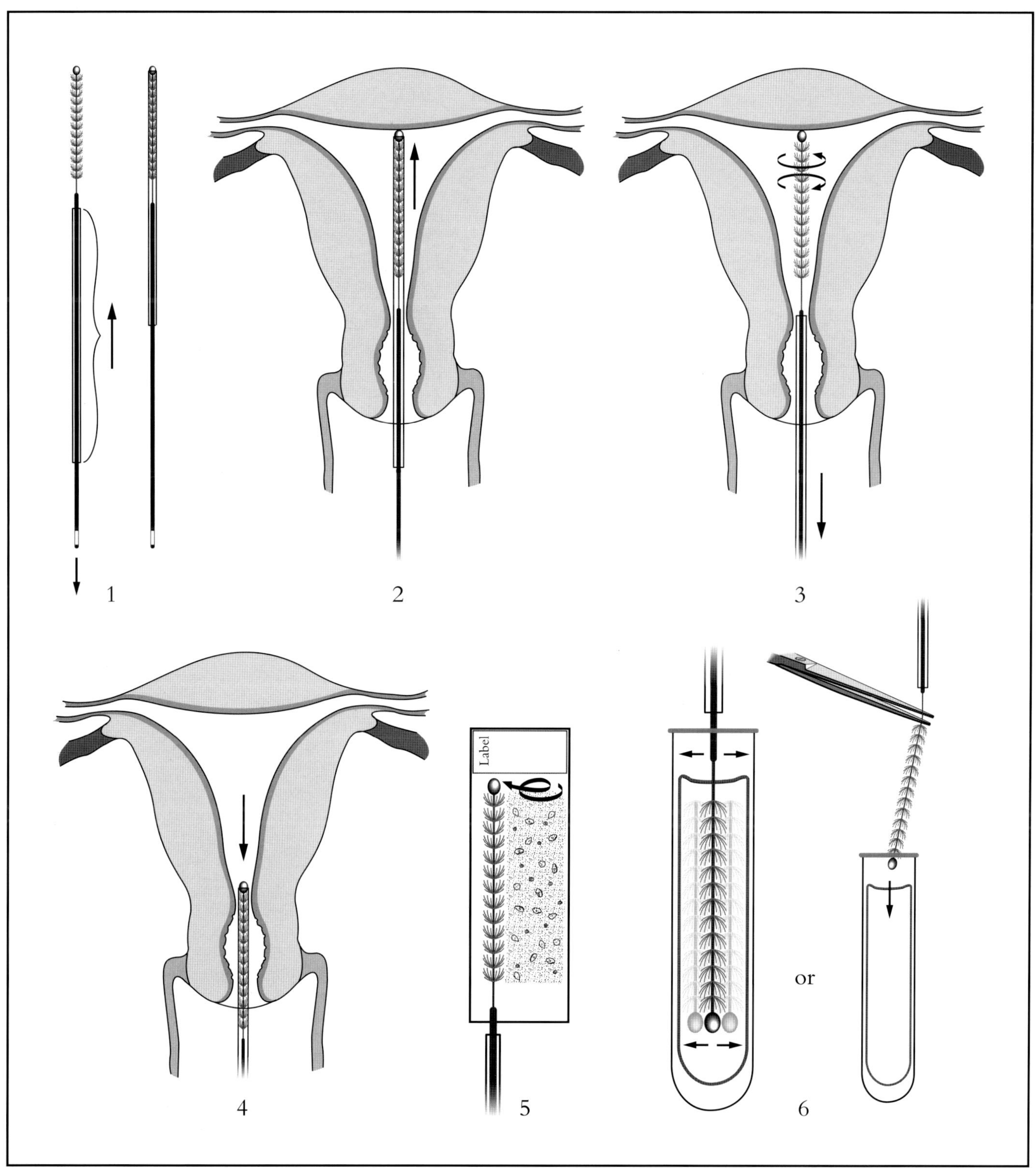

Figure 1.1 The procedure of endometrial sampling using the IUMC Endometrial Sampler. (1) Retract brush sampler completely into the outer tube. (2) Gently insert the device to the level of fundus. (3) Pull back outer tube to the level of internal os. Rotate brush sampler as it is withdrawn into the outer tube. (4) When the brush is retracted into the outer tube, remove the device. (5) Pull back outer tube, prepare a direct smear, and spray-fix immediately. (6) The material still attached to the brush is retrieved by shaking it in cytologic preservative or by cutting off the brush and dropping it into a container. *Note*: The normal endometrial cavity is in a collapsed state; thus, the brush has direct contact with the entire endometrial surface.

3. This cytologic technique does not interfere with subsequent histologic studies of the lesion when the cytologic findings are not diagnostic. One does not observe the disturbing changes that are inevitably present after curettage.
4. This cytologic technique provides enough material for cytomorphologic studies, even in asymptomatic patients for whom curettage is not indicated.

It is, therefore, an excellent technique for early detection of endometrial carcinoma and its precursors. Since this technique procures cells directly from the endometrial cavity, endometrial cells obtained are usually less degenerated (often well-preserved) than the corresponding cells seen in the cervicovaginal smears. In addition, the endometrial cells are more concentrated from this area, enabling accurate interpretation of endometrial pathology with proper training. This is a case-finding procedure, and we believe that family physicians should and can play an important role in screening patients for endometrial cancer. A previous knowledge of intrauterine device insertion is all that is required; in fact, the IUMC Endometrial Sampler has a smaller diameter and should be easier to use than the instruments employed for inserting intrauterine contraceptive devices.

Applications of Endometrial Cytology

This is a case-finding procedure for occult endometrial carcinoma and its precursors. In general, applications of endometrial cytology using this sampling device include:

1. Screening of patients at risk for endometrial carcinoma (eg, obese, diabetic, nulliparous, and hypertensive postmenopausal women).
2. Follow-up of patients receiving estrogen replacement therapy.
3. Follow-up of treated and untreated patients with endometrial hyperplasia.
4. Evaluation of postmenopausal women whose cervicovaginal smears show a high estrogen effect and/or endometrial cells.
5. Evaluation of patients with postmenopausal bleeding or other signs and symptoms warranting investigation of uterine pathology.

Koss et al[21] studied the results of screening of 2,586 asymptomatic women for occult endometrial carcinoma using Isaacs Endometrial Cell Sampler and Mi-Mark Helix techniques and found an incidence of 6.9 per 1,000. They concluded that the frequency of occult endometrial carcinoma warrants screening, and proposed that all women 50 years or older should have screening at least once. The incidence rate of 1.71 per 1,000 found on follow-up of 1 to 3 years was too small to justify the expense of a second screening.[21] Since experience in endometrial cytology is still being accumulated and there is a shortage of skilled manpower, a conservative approach should be considered. Screening every 3 years following a negative sample appears reasonable.

Table 1.3
Cytologic Interpretation of Endometrial Preparations★

1. No abnormal cells identified:
    a) Proliferative phase
    b) Secretory phase
    c) Menstrual phase
    d) Inactive endometrium
    e) Other ________________

2. Cellular changes consistent with:
    a) Acute endometritis
    b) Chronic endometritis
    c) Granulomatous endometritis
    d) Squamous metaplasia
    e) Irradiation changes
    f) Other ________________

3. Atypical cells consistent with endometrial hyperplasia:
    a) Mild
    b) Moderate
    c) Severe

4. Malignant cells consistent with:
    a) Adenocarcinoma
    b) Adenocarcinoma with squamous differentiation
    c) Clear cell carcinoma
    d) Stromal sarcoma
    e) Leiomyosarcoma
    f) Mixed müllerian tumor
    g) Other ________________

5. Atypical cells not specifically classified (see comments):

★This table represents an outline of what endometrial cytology (by direct intrauterine sampling) can demonstrate. It needs appropriate additional patient history and clinical data for it to be a complete form.

Since this technique is a simple, safe office procedure, it can also be used as a first-step examination by family physicians to assess post-menopausal bleeding. From the literature, only 5% to 15% of the cases of postmenopausal bleeding are due to endometrial carcinoma.[24,26] If any attempt using direct endometrial cytologic sampling is unsuccessful due to technical or diagnostic problems, dilation and curettage is warranted. Use of cytologic devices would result in a considerable monetary saving by decreasing the number of dilation and curettage procedures in those patients in whom there is no clinical suspicion of endometrial carcinoma and the endometrial cytology is negative. In Norway, Iversen and Segadal[16] use endometrial cytology as the first diagnostic procedure to assess postmenopausal bleeding, and have reduced curettage by 70 percent. In the United States approximately 210,000 dilation and curettage procedures are done every year.[22] With a dilation and curettage cost of $1,925, a 70% reduction would save $283 million in medical care costs.[17]

Although this technique is intended for early detection of endometrial carcinoma and its precursors, it can also be considered for clinical use in the following settings:

1. There are contraindications to perform a curettage (eg, cannot perform general anesthesia).
2. The patient does not permit a curettage.
3. The curettage does not yield sufficient diagnostic material (eg, a small lesion in a lateral cornu, which can be reached by means of an endometrial brush).

In a review of the different methods of screening for endometrial cancer, Boone et al[4] encouraged family physicians to use the new cytologic screening methods in view of their good yield, low cost, ease of use, and absence of major complications. Since the accuracy of cytomorphologic interpretation plays a major role in the success of this new technique, adequate training in endometrial cytology as well as a full awareness of the pitfalls in the interpretation are essential.

Although this technique is originally designed for the early detection of endometrial adenocarcinoma and its precursors, it can be used for diagnosing other cancers and benign disorders involving the endometrium. Cytomorphologic differentiation between proliferative phase and secretory phase endometria is also possible. This is discussed in the following chapters. A proposed report form for the cytologic interpretation of endometrial preparations is shown in Table 1.3.

References

1. Bamford DS, Hall EW, Newman MR: The Isaac endometrial cell sampler: An evaluation in 100 patients with postmenopausal bleeding. *Acta Cytol* 28:101–104, 1984.

2. Barbaro CA, Fortune DW, Bodey AS, et al: Uterine lavage in the diagnosis of endometrial malignancy and its precursors. *Acta Cytol* 26:135–140, 1982.

3. Beckner ME, Mori T, Silverberg SG: Endometrial carcinoma: Nontumor factors in prognosis. *Int J Gynecol Pathol* 4:131–145, 1985.

4. Boone MI, Calvert JC, Gates HS: Uterine cancer screening by the family physician. *Am Fam Physician* 30:157–166, 1984.

5. Buratti E, Cefis F, Masserini M, et al: The value of endometrial cytology in a high risk population. *Tumori* 71:25–28, 1985.

6. *Cancer Facts and Figures—1992*. Atlanta, American Cancer Society, 1992, p 5.

7. Costa MM, Einhorn N, Sjovall K, et al: Endometrial carcinoma diagnosed by the Gynoscan method. *Acta Obstet Gynecol Scand* 65:473–475, 1986.

8. Cramer JH, Osborne RJ: Endometrial neoplasia: Screening of high risk patient. *Am J Obstet Gynecol* 139:285–288, 1981.

9. Crow J, Gordon H, Hudson E: An assessment of the Mi-Mark endometrial sampler technique. *J Clin Pathol* 33:72–80, 1980.

10. Deligdisch L, Cohen CJ: Histologic correlates and virulence implications of endometrial carcinoma associated with adenomatous hyperplasia. *Cancer* 56:1452–1455, 1985.

11. Elwood MJ, Cole P, Rothman KJ, et al: Epidemiology of endometrial cancer. *J Natl Cancer Inst* 59:1055–1060, 1977.

12. Ferenczy A, Gelfland MM: Outpatient endometrial sampling with endocyte: Comparative study of its effectiveness with endometrial biopsy. *Obstet Gynecol* 63:295–302, 1984.

13. Fox H, Sen DK: A controlled study of the constitutional stigmata of endometrial adenocarcinoma. *Br J Cancer* 24:30–36, 1970.

14. Inoue Y, Ikeda M, Kimura K, et al: Accuracy of endometrial aspiration in the diagnosis of endometrial cancer. *Acta Cytol* 27:477–481, 1983.

15. Isaacs JH, Wilhoite RW: Aspiration cytology of the endometrium: Office and hospital sampling procedures. *Am J Obstet Gynecol* 118:679–687, 1974.

16. Iversen OE, Segadal E: The value of endometrial cytology: A comparative study of the Gravlee Jet-Washing, Isaacs Cell Sampler, and Endoscann versus curettage in 600 patients. *Obstet Gynecol Surv* 40:14–20, 1985.

17. Jaber R: Detection of and screening for endometrial cancer. *J Fam Pract* 26:67–72, 1988.

18. Judd HL, Davidson BJ, Frumar AM, et al: Serum androgens in postmenopausal women with and without endometrial cancer. *Am J Obstet Gynecol* 136:859–871, 1980.

19. Koss LG, Schreiber K, Moussouris H, et al: Endometrial carcinoma and its precursors: Detection and screening. *Clin Obstet Gynecol* 25:49–61, 1982.

20. Koss LG, Schreiber K, Oberlander SG, et al: Screening of asymptomatic women for endometrial cancer. *Obstet Gynecol* 57:681–691, 1981.

21. Koss LG, Schreiber K, Oberlander SG, et al: Detection of endometrial carcinoma and hyperplasia in asymptomatic women. *Obstet Gynecol* 64:1–11, 1984.

22. Kozak LJ, Moien M: Detailed diagnoses and surgical procedures for patients discharged from short stay hospitals: United States, 1983. In: *National Center for Health Statistics. Vital and Health Statistics.* Series 13, No. 82. Washington, Government Printing Office, 1985, p 173. Department of Health and Human Services Publication No. 86-1743.

23. Kriseman MM: Description of a new disposable uterine sampler (the Accuratte) for endometrial cytology and histology. *S Afr Med J* 61:107–108, 1981.

24. McElin TW, Bird CC, Reeves BD, et al: Diagnostic dilation and curettages: A 20-year survey. *Obstet Gynecol* 33:807–812, 1969.

25. Meisels A, Fortier M, Jolicoeus C: Endometrial hyperplasia and neoplasia: Cytologic screening with Endo-Pap endometrial sampler. *J Reprod Med* 28:309–313, 1983.

26. Pacheco JC, Kempers RD: Etiology of postmenopausal bleeding. *Obstet Gynecol* 32:40–46, 1968.

27. Palermo V: Interpretation of endometrium obtained by the Endo-Pap sampler and a clinical study of its use. *Diagn Cytopathol* 1:5–12, 1985.

28. Palermo VG: The detection of endometrial adenocarcinoma using the Endo-Pap endometrial cytology sampler. *Acta Cytol* 26:738, 1982.

29. Palermo VG, Blythe JG, Kaufman RH: Cytologic diagnosis of endometrial adenocarcinoma using the Endo-Pap sampler. *Obstet Gynecol* 65:271–275, 1985.

30. Reagan JW: Can screening for endometrial cancer be justified? *Acta Cytol* 24:87–89, 1980.

31. Segadal E, Iversen OE: Endoscann, a new endometrial cell sampler. *Br J Obstet Gynecol* 90:266–271, 1983.

32. Siiteri PK: Steroid hormones and endometrial cancer. *Cancer Res* 38:4360–4366, 1978.

33. Silverberg SG, Makowski EL, Roche WD: Endometrial carcinoma in women under 40 years of age. *Cancer* 39:592–598, 1977.

34. Silverberg SG, Mullen D, Faraci JA, et al: Endometrial carcinoma: Clinical-pathologic comparison of cases in postmenopausal women receiving and not receiving exogenous estrogens. *Cancer* 45:3018–3026, 1980.

35. Veneti SZ, Kyrkou KA, Kittas CN, et al: Efficacy of the Isaacs endometrial cell sampler in the cytologic detection of endometrial abnormalities. *Acta Cytol* 28:546–556, 1984.

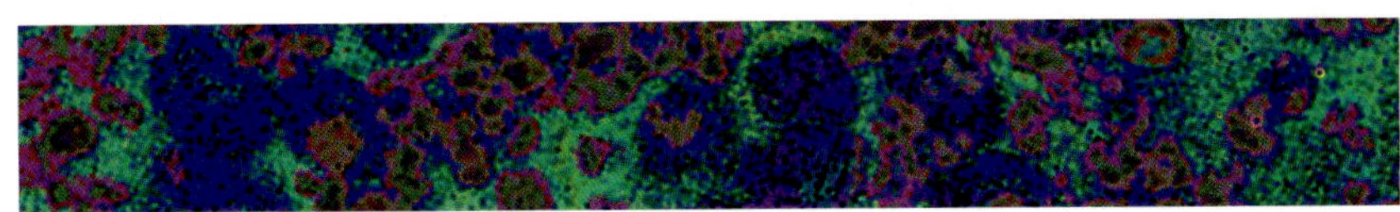

CHAPTER TWO

Cytology of the Normal Endometrium

Endometrial cytology has been the focus of great interest in part due to rising incidence of endometrial adenocarcinoma. The success of Papanicolaou smears in the early detection of cervical carcinoma and its precursors has also given hope for the early detection of endometrial carcinoma and its precursors. However, endometrial smears are more difficult to interpret than cervicovaginal smears.[5,11,12,16] Both endometrial glandular and stromal cells undergo cyclic changes, and their cytomorphologic appearances vary greatly at different stages of the cycle. The appearance of normal endometrial cells is related to many factors, such as the site of origin in the endometrium, the stage of the menstrual cycle, the administration of estrogen and/or progesterone, and the method used to collect the endometrial sample.[18] In addition, the cytomorphologic differences among proliferative glandular cells, hyperplastic glandular cells, and well-differentiated neoplastic glandular cells are very subtle.[11,12]

It is not unusual for pathologists to make mistakes in the interpretation of endometrial cytologic preparations or sign out too many "suspicious" reports. This is due mainly to the fact that they lack the special training needed to become familiar with the cytomorphologic appearances of the endometrial glandular and stromal cells during different stages of the menstrual cycle, and with the cytologic features of different types of lesions in endometrial cytologic preparations, which have markedly different morphologic appearances from those seen on tissue sections.

The Uterine Mucosa

The adult uterus consists of a body, the corpus, and a smaller cervix. The fundus is the portion of the corpus cephalad to a line connecting the origin of two fallopian tubes. The cornua are the two lateral regions of the fundus associated with the intramural portion of the fallopian tubes. The remainder of the body tapers from the fundus into the lower uterine segment, which shares histologic features with both the uterine corpus and the endocervix. The endometrial cavity is triangular and the apices of this potential space are continuous with the lumina of the fallopian tubes at the two cornua and with the endocervical canal at the internal os. The transition from endometrial cavity to endocervix is gradual without abrupt anatomic demarcation. This is histologically mirrored by the gradual transition of the mucosa in this region from endometrial type to endocervical type.

The uterine mucosa can be divided into two regions: the mucosa of the lower uterine segment (isthmus) and the mucosa of the corpus proper. The mucosa of the isthmus, located between endocervix and endometrium, is generally thinner than that of the fundus. The glands and stroma in this region are only sluggishly responsive to hormonal stimulation. The morphologic transition from mucosa of the isthmus to endocervical mucosa is gradual, and there is a hybrid endometrial-endocervical appearance of both the glands and the stroma of the isthmus.

The major portion of the uterine mucosa, the corpus endometrium proper, is fully responsive to hormonal stimulation. Two layers can be readily identified within the endometrium in this region: the lowermost is called the basalis and the overlying one the functionalis (Images 2.1 and 2.2). The basalis is the inactive zone immediately adjacent to the myometrium and consists of weakly proliferative glands and dense spindled stroma. The appearance of the basalis is relatively constant throughout the menstrual cycle. It constitutes the "reserve cell layer" of the endometrium. After the bulk of the functionalis is shed during menstruation, or after the functionalis is removed by curettage, the basalis and the residual deep functionalis are responsible for regenerating the endometrium.

Cellular Components of the Endometrium

During the reproductive years the normal endometrium consists of glandular epithelia (proliferative, secretory, and surface glandular epithelia), and stromal and vascular elements. They first synchronously proliferate, then differentiate, and finally disintegrate at roughly 28-day intervals. During a 28-day cycle, proliferation is the dominant reaction in the endometrium from days 4 to 13 (proliferative phase). As the proliferative phase advances, the endometrium increases in thickness and the glands become more tortuous and have more dilated lumina. The intervening stromal cells are enlarged or may be altered by transient edema. After ovulation occurs secretion is present in the epithelium of the endometrium. This is designated as the secretory phase (days 14–28). This change usually becomes evident on day 16. At this time, the endometrium is thick with closely spaced tortuous glands having dilated lumina. Prior to menstruation there is a sudden reduction in the thickness of the endometrium due to a decrease in ovarian steroids. This reduction in thickness impairs the blood flow to the upper portion of the endometrium, resulting in ischemia leading to necrosis and hemorrhage. During a menstrual cycle the glandular epithelium lining the glands and intervening stromal cells undergo morphologic changes, whereas the surface glandular epithelium and glandular and stromal elements in the basalis and in the lower uterine segment show no significant morphologic changes.

The Epithelial Cells of the Endometrium

The endometrial glandular and surface epithelia are composed of three morphologically distinct cells, namely, proliferative glandular and basalis glandular cells, secretory glandular cells, and ciliated glandular cells.

Proliferative Glandular Cells

The proliferative glandular cells of the functionalis and glandular cells of the basalis are morphologically quite similar. In endometrial brushing preparations, these cells both have scant cytoplasm and round, ovoid, or slightly elongated nuclei with dense chromatin and inconspicuous or small nucleoli. They usually occur in sheets or cohesive groupings because of the inherent mutual adhesiveness between glandular cells. The cytoplasmic boundaries are ill-defined. Nuclear crowding and overlapping are apparent, and mitotic figures are common in the glandular and stromal cells of the functionalis during the proliferative phase (Images 2.3 and 2.4). In general, early proliferative glandular cells show relatively little evidence of estrogenic stimulation, whereas those in the midproliferative and late proliferative phases show increasing degrees of stratification, mitotic activity, nuclear enlargement, and nucleolar prominence.

Secretory Glandular Cells

Soon after ovulation, secretory products accumulate in a subnuclear location, gradually shift to a supranuclear position, and are ultimately discharged into the glandular lumens. In endometrial brushing preparations from secretory endometrium during the ovulatory phase, the glandular cells have small, round or ovoid nuclei with dense chromatin and inconspicuous or small nucleoli and an increased amount of cytoplasm (as compared with that of the proliferative glandular cells). Some of the glandular cells with partially perinuclear clearing of the cytoplasm intermix with glandular cells with dense cytoplasm (Image 2.5).

During early and midsecretory phases, the glandular cells have clear cytoplasm and well-demarcated cytoplasmic boundaries in endometrial brushing preparations. During the early secretory phase, the secretory glandular cells have round or ovoid nuclei with dense chromatin and inconspicuous or small nucleoli similar to those of the glandular cells seen during the proliferative phase (Image 2.6), whereas during the midsecretory phase the secretory glandular cells have enlarged, rounded and vesicular nuclei with uniformly dispersed chromatin and occasional small or prominent nucleoli. The secretory glandular cells during the midsecretory phase are larger than those during the early secretory phase, and have a moderate amount of well-defined, clear cytoplasm. They are in sheet arrangements with a honeycomb pattern (Image 2.7).

During the late secretory phase, some of the glandular cells have smaller, round or ovoid nuclei with slightly coarse or coarse chromatin and a moderate amount of well-defined, somewhat dense cytoplasm in endometrial brushing preparations. They are also in sheet arrangements and probably represent "exhausted" secretory glandular cells (Image 2.8). However, if implantation of a blastocyst occurs, the glandular cells become "exaggerated" secretory cells during early pregnancy. They have an abundance of well-defined, clear cytoplasm and enlarged, round or ovoid, vesicular nuclei. They also occur in sheet arrangements with a honeycomb pattern (Image 2.9). After the cessation of menstrual periods, the menopause begins and the endometrium becomes atrophic. The glandular cells have small, round or ovoid, dense or pyknotic nuclei and scant, nonvacuolated cytoplasm. They remain in sheet arrangements (Image 2.10).

Ciliated Glandular Cells

The ciliated glandular cells are consistently present in the endometrium and frequently seen in endometrial specimens. Their presence in the endometrium illustrates the ability of endometrial glandular cells to differentiate along the lines of other normal müllerian tissues (tubal or endocervical). These cells are more prominent near the uterine isthmus and readily identified in regenerated epithelium during the proliferative phase.[4,10,19] They may also be noticed during the secretory phase. They occur more often in estrogen-stimulated endometria. They have well-developed cilia over their free margins, and have centrally placed, ovoid, smoothly contoured vesicular nuclei with finely stippled chromatin. The size of the ciliated glandular cells is often smaller than that of the secretory glandular cells seen during the midsecretory or late secretory phase. They are columnar cells in palisading arrangements and often contain brightly eosinophilic cytoplasm (Images 2.11 and 2.12). Tubal, ciliated, or eosinophilic metaplasia has been used to describe the presence of these cells in large numbers.

The Stromal Cells of the Endometrium

In endometrial brushing preparations, the appearance of the endometrial stromal cells varies greatly with the stage of the menstrual cycle. During the early proliferative phase, the stromal cells have scant, ill-defined cytoplasm and ovoid or fusiform nuclei, and occur singly or in loose groupings (Image 2.13). As the menstrual cycle proceeds, the stromal cells that have ovoid or fusiform nuclei become spindled and acquire more cytoplasm. During the late proliferative and early secretory phases, there is a peripheral condensation of their cytoplasm, and the spindled stromal cells often occur in cohesive groups (Image 2.14). During the midsecretory phase, the stromal cells have enlarged, plump, vesicular nuclei and scant, ill-defined cytoplasm (Image 2.15).

During the late secretory phase, the stromal cells in the upper portion of the endometrium undergo predecidual changes associated with an increased glycogen content. They acquire abundant cytoplasm with relatively well-demarcated cytoplasmic boundaries, and contain large, round or ovoid, vesicular nuclei with occasional prominent nucleoli.[10] The nuclei of predecidual cells (the predecidualized stromal cells) are usually centrally located. In endometrial brushing preparations from endometrium of the late secretory phase, the stromal cells exhibit varying degrees of predecidualization, from small stromal cells (from the lower portion of the endometrium), to large predecidualized stromal cells (from the upper portion of the endometrium), to very large ones with large nuclei and prominent nucleoli (from the perivascular regions, seen on the last 2 days of the menstrual cycle), resembling decidual cells seen during pregnancy (Images 2.16–2.22).

During the menstrual phase, the stroma disintegrates and many predecidual cells in the upper portion of the endometrium separate from each other and become rounded. They are seen in the endometrial cavity in large numbers. They have round, ovoid, or bean-shaped nuclei and various amounts of relatively well-defined, foamy or finely granular cytoplasm morphologically mimicking histiocytes. Cytoplasmic vacuoles are noted in some of these cells and often contain neutrophils (Image 2.23). These solitary predecidual cells may also be seen as an exodus of histiocyte-like cells in cervicovaginal smears procured during or shortly after the menstrual phase.

During early pregnancy the predecidual cells are gradually converted to decidual cells. These enlarged decidualized stromal cells have large vesicular nuclei and an abundance of well-defined, clear or foamy cytoplasm due to the increased intracytoplasmic glycogen. They occur in sheet arrangements or in loose or cohesive groupings (Image 2.24).

After the menopause, atrophy of the endometrium proceeds progressively, and the stromal cells become spindled and are closely packed. They have scant, ill-defined cytoplasm and plump, fusiform or pyknotic nuclei (Image 2.25).

The stromal foam cells (Images 2.26–2.32) are a special type of stromal cell often seen in patients with endometrial adenocarcinoma or endometrial hyperplasia. These cells are rarely observed in benign conditions of the endometrium, therefore their presence serves to warn of endometrial hyperplasia or carcinoma. These cells have relatively large, centrally placed, ovoid nuclei with small nucleoli and fine chromatin. They have an abundance of foamy cytoplasm, which is rich in lipids (neutral fats). Similar cells with clear cytoplasm, probably resulting from the fusion of lipid vacuoles, are also seen.

The stromal foam cells are relatively uniform in size, and often occur in cohesive clusters. These cytologic features distinguish them from morphologically similar foamy histiocytes that virtually always occur singly in endometrial brushing preparations. Foamy histiocytes have well-defined, foamy or vacuolated cytoplasm and ovoid or bean-shaped nuclei, often peripherally located (Image 2.33). They are variable in size and are encountered in conditions with tissue breakdown or inflammation, after the injection of contrast medium, or in endometrium of the late secretory or menstrual phase. They are usually present in the lumina of glands or the endometrial cavity, rather than in stroma. The stromal foam cells are only present in stroma of the endometria (not seen in the lumina of endometrial glands) constantly stimulated by estrogen, and are thought to be of stromal rather than histiocytic origin.[2,3]

In endometrial brushing preparations, one may find transitional-type cells with less abundant, finely granular cytoplasm morphologically between stromal foam cells and regular stromal cells. The finding of stromal foam cells admixed with regular stromal cells in the same cell clusters also substantiates the view that these foam cells are of stromal origin. An ultrastructural study has likewise shown that they are altered endometrial stromal cells.[6] In fact, the recognition of true stromal foam cells (not foamy histiocytes) in endometrial brushing preparations is helpful in diagnosing well-differentiated adenocarcinoma or endometrial hyperplasia.

In endometrial brushing preparations, smooth muscle cells from the myometrium are occasionally encountered. The cytologic appearance of uterine smooth muscle cells differs substantially from that of the endometrial stromal cells present in the proliferative or early to midsecretory phase endometrium. However, groups of stromal cells with predecidual changes (predecidual cells that have enlarged, round or ovoid nuclei and abundant cytoplasm) seen during the late secretory phase may resemble smooth muscle cells in endometrial brushing preparations, in which smooth muscle cells occur in cohesive groupings with loosely and somewhat regularly arranged nuclei. The smooth muscle cells have ovoid, spindle-shaped, or blunt-ended elongated nuclei with a fine chromatin pattern, and abundant cytoplasm with ill-defined cellular boundaries, often appearing in syncytial arrangements (Images 2.34 and 2.35). In contrast, the stromal cells with predecidual changes usually have round or ovoid nuclei with frequent small or prominent nucleoli and relatively well-defined cellular boundaries within cell clusters.

Cyclic Morphologic Changes of the Endometrium

The endometrium undergoes cyclic morphologic changes that are particularly striking during the reproductive years and are characterized by regularly occurring, roughly monthly cycles, the end of which is signaled by menstrual bleeding.[7,9] During the first half of the menstrual cycle the ovarian-secreted estradiol induces endometrial proliferation. The second half of the cycle is hormonally dominated by both estradiol and progesterone, which induce endometrial glandular secretion and stromal predecidualization. With the withdrawal of corpus luteum steroidal support, the endometrium is shed, setting the stage for the next cycle. The menstrual cycle is divided into three phases, each of which is associated with characteristic endometrial morphologic features that are described below.

The endometrium undergoes three major phases of cyclic morphologic changes

The Proliferative Phase
The endometrium responds to rising estrogen levels by synchronous proliferation of glands, stroma, and blood vessels. During the early proliferative phase (the first third after menstruation, or days 4–7), the rate of growth of all three elements is coordinated. Both glands and blood vessels are straight. The glands have regular contours, are of small diameter, and

are dispersed in a relatively dense stroma. During the midproliferative and late proliferative phases, the growth of both glands and blood vessels outstrips that of the stroma, and as a result they become coiled. The nuclei of glandular cells become slightly elongated and are found at the base of the cell. The stroma is abundant and dense. Moderate to marked stromal edema may be seen during the midproliferative phase.

During the late proliferative phase, the glands are lined by pseudostratified or stratified columnar cells with high nuclear/cytoplasmic ratios and dense chromatin. Small or prominent nucleoli may be seen. Mitotic figures are easy to find. After day 11, scattered small subnuclear vacuoles begin to appear, resulting from the accumulation of glycogen inclusions at the base of the glandular cells. Their identity as glycogen may be confirmed by a periodic acid–Schiff (PAS) stain. During the last 2 days of the proliferative phase mitotic figures are infrequent, glandular coiling becomes more prominent, and scattered small subnuclear vacuoles are easy to find. The gland contours become more sinuous and their diameters increase as well. The stromal edema may be present.

In endometrial brushing preparations from the proliferative phase endometrium, the proliferative glandular cells have scant cytoplasm and have ovoid nuclei with dense chromatin and inconspicuous or small nucleoli. They occur in cohesive, sheet arrangements with nuclear crowding and overlapping against a relatively clean background. During the early proliferative phase, segments of straight, tubular glands are often seen. The stromal cells that have scant, ill-defined cytoplasm and ovoid or fusiform nuclei occur singly or in loose, noncohesive groupings (Images 2.36–2.39). The cytologic findings during the midproliferative phase are similar to those seen during the early proliferative phase except that there are no straight, tubular glands and the glandular cells often show small nucleoli. The stromal cells in the midproliferative phase acquire more cytoplasm, become spindled, and occur in loose or cohesive groupings (Images 2.40–2.42). During the late proliferative phase, occasional glandular cells with partially perinuclear clearing (corresponding to small subnuclear vacuoles seen on histologic sections) are seen. The spindled stromal cells that have an abundance of ill-defined cytoplasm occur in loose or cohesive groupings (Images 2.43–2.47).

The Secretory Phase

The morphologic changes during the secretory phase of a 28-day cycle can be divided into four periods: ovulatory (days 14 and 15), early secretory (days 16–19), midsecretory (days 20–23), and late secretory (days 24–28). In the first 36 to 48 hours of the secretory phase, the endometrium for the most part retains its late proliferative phase appearance morphologically, although more small subnuclear vacuoles are usually seen. This morphologically indeterminate endometrium is termed ovulatory phase.

The first unequivocal light microscopic indication that ovulation has occurred is the presence of numerous large, well-developed subnuclear vacuoles and nuclear palisading involving more than 50% of the endometrial glands—a finding typical of day 17. Over the next 2 days, these vacuoles shift from a subnuclear to a supranuclear location. By the fifth postovulatory day, most of the secretion has been discharged into the glandular lumen. The morphologic hallmark of the early secretory phase is the vacuolated glandular cells that retain small, ovoid nuclei with dense chromatin, as seen in the proliferative phase endometrium. Scattered mitotic figures may be found. The stromal cells are spindled and have the same appearance as they had during the late proliferative phase.

The midsecretory phase is characterized by prominently coiled secretory glands containing abundant luminal secretion and set within an edematous stroma. The glandular cells appear nonvacuolated on histologic sections by hematoxylin-eosin stain, and have enlarged, round, somewhat vesicular nuclei. However, the cytoplasm of glandular cells, unlike what is seen on histologic sections, appears clear in endometrial brushing preparations by Papanicolaou stain.

The characteristic features of the late secretory phase are stromal pre-decidualization and an increased prominence of the spiral arteries. The secretory glands begin to show regressive changes related to the decreasing level of circulating progesterone. By day 24, cuffs or islands of predecidual cells are present around these spiral arteries near the surface of the endometrium. Over the next 3 days, these islands become confluent, and stromal infiltration by neutrophils and endometrial granulocytes is noted. The intensity of this infiltration is closely correlated with the time of onset of menses. The endometrial granulocytes are only seen during the last week of the menstrual cycle. They resemble lymphocytes but have a rim of cytoplasm containing granules that are thought to represent a substance called relaxin. The function of relaxin is to dissolve the reticulin fibers sur-rounding individual stromal cells, thus allowing the stromal cells to disso-ciate and normal menstrual shedding to take place. The glandular appear-ance during the late secretory phase is not significantly different from its appearance during the midsecretory phase on histologic sections; but in endometrial brushing preparations, the cytoplasm of some of the secretory glandular cells seen during the late secretory phase are partially clear or not clear and appear somewhat dense, and the nuclei of some glandular cells are slightly smaller and appear dense.

In endometrial brushing preparations from the secretory phase endometrium there is some mucoid material in the background (best seen in direct smears), which usually becomes evident after day 16. Dur-ing the ovulatory period (days 14 and 15), the glandular and stromal cells have a morphologic appearance similar to that of the late proliferative phase, except that the glandular cells are less crowded and there are more glandular cells with partially perinuclear clearing intermixed with glan-dular cells with dense cytoplasm. The background is relatively clean or slightly mucoid. Therefore, the characteristic feature of the ovulatory phase in endometrial brushing preparations is the presence of a mixture of proliferative glandular cells and secretory glandular cells with partially perinuclear clearing, in sheet arrangements without significant nuclear crowding and overlapping (Images 2.48–2.51).

As the secretory phase progresses, the glandular cells become larger and contain an increased amount of well-defined, clear cytoplasm. They are in sheet arrangements with a honeycomb pattern. There is more mucoid material in the background. During the early secretory phase, the glandular cells have round or ovoid nuclei with dense chromatin and conspicuous or small nucleoli. The spindled stromal cells have an abun-dance of ill-defined cytoplasm and ovoid or fusiform nuclei with dense chromatin, and occur in loose or cohesive groupings (Images 2.52–2.55).

During the midsecretory phase, the cytoplasm of the glandular cells remains clear, but their nuclei become larger, rounded, and somewhat vesicular with a fine chromatin pattern and occasional small or prominent nucleoli. There is copious, thick mucoid material in the background. The stromal cells have scant, ill-defined cytoplasm and enlarged, plump, vesicular nuclei with fine chromatin. They occur singly or in loose, noncohesive groupings (Images 2.56–2.60).

During the late secretory phase, some of the glandular cells have smaller, round or ovoid nuclei with slightly coarse or coarse chromatin and a moderate amount of well-defined, somewhat dense cytoplasm. They probably represent "exhausted" secretory glandular cells. The stromal cells in the upper portion of the endometrium undergo predecidual changes, and the predecidual cells that have an abundance of relatively well-defined, dense cytoplasm and centrally located, round or ovoid, vesicular nuclei occur in sheet arrangements or in loose or cohesive groupings. Small or prominent nucleoli may be seen in some predecidual cells, and variations in cellular size and nuclear size are apparent in some groups of predecidual cells (Images 2.61–2.68). Increasing numbers of neutrophils and endometrial granulocytes are also noted.

At the end of the late secretory phase as the stroma begins to disintegrate, many predecidual cells in the upper portion of the endometrium separate from each other and are present in the endometrial cavity in large numbers. Thus, in endometrial brushing preparations there are numerous solitary predecidual cells with round, ovoid, or bean-shaped nuclei and various amounts of relatively well-defined, foamy or finely granular cytoplasm. Cytoplasmic vacuoles containing neutrophils may be seen in these solitary predecidual cells (Image 2.69). However, towards the end of the secretory phase, some of the perivascular predecidual cells become very large with large nuclei and frequent prominent nucleoli, resembling decidual cells seen during pregnancy. Their cytoplasm is usually denser than that of decidual cells. They may show nuclear pleomorphism and cytologic atypia.

If implantation of a blastocyst occurs during the midsecretory phase, it is associated with a resurgence of prominent glandular secretion and exaggerated stromal decidualization. Many of the glands are lined by enlarged glandular cells containing large nuclei with fine or slightly coarse chromatin and abundant clear cytoplasm. The developing predecidua of the late secretory phase is gradually converted to decidua. This transformation is generally complete by the end of the first month of gestation. Almost all of the endometrial stroma is converted into sheets or masses of very large decidual cells with well-defined cytoplasmic margins and large centrally located, vesicular nuclei. These changes may also be seen in the endometrium during ectopic pregnancy.

In endometrial brushing preparations, the predecidual cells normally seen during the late secretory phase do not separate from each other when implantation of a blastocyst occurs. They transform into very large decidual cells that have large vesicular nuclei with frequent prominent nucleoli and an abundance of well-defined, finely granular, foamy or clear cytoplasm due to the increased intracytoplasmic glycogen. They occur in sheet arrangements, or in loose or cohesive groupings. The secretory glandular cells also do not have the appearance of "exhausted" secretory glandular cells as normally seen during the late secretory phase.

Instead, they become "exaggerated" secretory glandular cells that have enlarged nuclei and an abundance of clear cytoplasm, and are larger (Images 2.70-2.73).

The Menstrual Phase

The imminent dissolution of the endometrium is first evidenced by the appearance of stromal hemorrhage and increased numbers of leukocytes. The functionalis undergoes shrinkage, and its constituent glands and stroma fragment and crumble. Fibrin thrombi appear in blood vessels and within the stroma.[14] As the stroma disintegrates, the glands are arranged randomly and come to lie close to one another. The endometrium contains collapsed stroma, ruptured glands, numerous solitary predecidual cells, neutrophils, endometrial granulocytes, and nuclear debris.

The endometrial brushing preparations are invariably bloody and inflamed, and contain menstrual detritus. There are many ball-like tissue fragments (or menstrual cell balls) consisting of closely packed, degenerating glandular cells and/or stromal cells intermixed with leukocytes and nuclear debris. Typically, in the center of menstrual cell balls are degenerating glandular cells surrounded by predecidual cells (from the upper portion of the endometrium) or rarely by small stromal cells (from the lower portion of the endometrium). These ball-like tissue fragments are only seen during the menstrual phase, thus this finding indicates a normal menstrual endometrium. Menstrual cell balls consisting only of predecidual cells admixed with leukocytes are also noted (Images 2.74–2.77). In addition, numerous predecidual cells occur as solitary cells or in loose groupings. They have round, ovoid, or bean-shaped nuclei with slightly coarse chromatin and various amounts of relatively well-defined, finely granular or foamy cytoplasm, resembling histiocytes. Cytoplasmic vacuolation is noted in some of the solitary predecidual cells. It is not uncommon to find neutrophils within the vacuoles. These solitary predecidual cells are also seen in cervicovaginal smears procured during or shortly after the menstrual phase, and appear as an exodus of histiocyte-like cells with accompanying menstrual detritus often containing menstrual cell balls (Image 2.78).

The Endometrium in Perimenopausal and Postmenopausal Women

The end of ovarian follicular development and ovulation results in cessation of the menstrual periods and the menopause. Thereafter, the uterus enters an inactive period and the endometrium becomes atrophic. Atrophy of the endometrium proceeds progressively after the menopause, and in some cases this transformation may take years.[17] This is why it is not rare to find signs of proliferative activity after the menopause. The existence of extraovarian sources of genital hormones, notably the adrenal cortices, explains the persistence of a certain degree of hormonal activity long after menopause. McBride[13] has shown in 1,521 cases of curettage in postmenopausal women that the endometrium was of the atrophic type in 31.5%; of the cystic atrophic type in 42.7%; and in 12.6%, who were only a few years postmenopausal, proliferative endometria were seen. The thickness of the endometrium and the glandular architecture may vary greatly. Several patterns may be seen in the perimenopausal and postmenopausal endometria.

The Atrophic Endometrium

The atrophic endometrium is thin and smooth. It measures about 0.4 mm in thickness. The endometrial glands in this condition comprise a single layer of flattened to cuboidal cells with scant, nonvacuolated cytoplasm and high nuclear/cytoplasmic ratio. The nuclei of glandular cells are small and ovoid, and may be pyknotic. Mitotic figures are not present. The glands of the atrophic endometrium may have various configurations, including cystic dilation and glandular crowding. The stromal cells are spindled and closely packed. They will not become predecidualized. Their nuclei are plump or fusiform and may be pyknotic. Atrophic endometrium can also occur in premenopausal women in association with premature ovarian failure or, more commonly, in women taking oral contraceptives or receiving continuous therapy with progestational agents.[1,15] In the latter conditions, the endometrial glands are small and appear inactive, but the cytoplasm of the stromal cells becomes more abundant and dense, reminiscent of predecidual or decidual changes seen during the late secretory phase or early pregnancy.

In endometrial brushing preparations from the atrophic endometrium, the specimen is often scantily cellular and contains a few sheets of glandular cells and several groups of spindle stromal cells. The glandular cells that have relatively small, round or ovoid, dense or pyknotic nuclei and scant cytoplasm occur in sheet arrangements. Nuclear crowding and overlapping are not seen. The stromal cells that have ovoid, fusiform, or pyknotic nuclei occur in loose groupings (Images 2.79–2.83). In endometrial brushing preparations from women taking oral contraceptives or progestational agents for a prolonged period, the glandular cells are similar to those seen in postmenopausal atrophic endometrium; however, the stromal cells appear different and contain a moderate amount of somewhat dense cytoplasm and large vesicular nuclei, resembling predecidual or decidual cells (Images 2.84 and 2.85).

The Weakly Proliferative Endometrium

Weakly proliferative endometria are encountered most often in perimenopausal or postmenopausal women whose endometria are weakly supported by low levels of endogenous or exogenous estrogen. This pattern is essentially the same as that in the hormonally hyporesponsive lower uterine segment of normally cycling premenopausal women. The glandular epithelium is nonstratified, although some degree of nuclear pseudostratification may be present. The glandular cells are thin columnar or cuboidal cells and have a dense nucleus. Mitotic figures are scarce. The glands may be of any configuration, but the glands-to-stroma ratio is near unity. The stomal cells are spindled, and their nuclei are plump or fusiform and may be pyknotic.

In endometrial brushing preparations from the weakly proliferative endometrium, the glandular cells are similar to those seen during the early proliferative phase, except that the nuclei appear less crowded and mitotic figures are scarce. The stromal cells are fibroblast-like, and their nuclei are plump or fusiform and may be pyknotic (Images 2.86–2.89).

The Disordered Proliferative Endometrium

This pattern is encountered in women with sporadic anovulatory cycles and thus is seen in the perimenopausal years. It is also seen in women receiving estrogen therapy. It probably represents the response of a normal endometrium to sporadic unopposed estrogen stimulation.[8] Disordered proliferative endometrium differs from normal proliferative phase endometrium by virtue of a loss of synchrony of glandular development so that some glands are tubular and others are cystically dilated or have complex shapes.[8] Budding may be present. There may be a slight shift in the glands-to-stroma ratio in favor of the glands. The variously shaped glands are lined by normal proliferative glandular cells with ovoid or elongated nuclei and dense chromatin. Pseudostratification of the glandular epithelial cells and mitotic figures are present. The stromal cells are spindled and have plump nuclei. In endometrial brushing preparations, the cytologic findings are essentially the same as those seen in endometrium of the proliferative phase during the reproductive years (Images 2.90–2.93).

Image 2.1
Functionalis and basalis of the endometrium. Two layers can be identified within the endometrium: the lowermost is the basalis and the overlying one the functionalis. The basalis is relatively constant throughout the menstrual cycle. Histologic section (H&E, 40X).

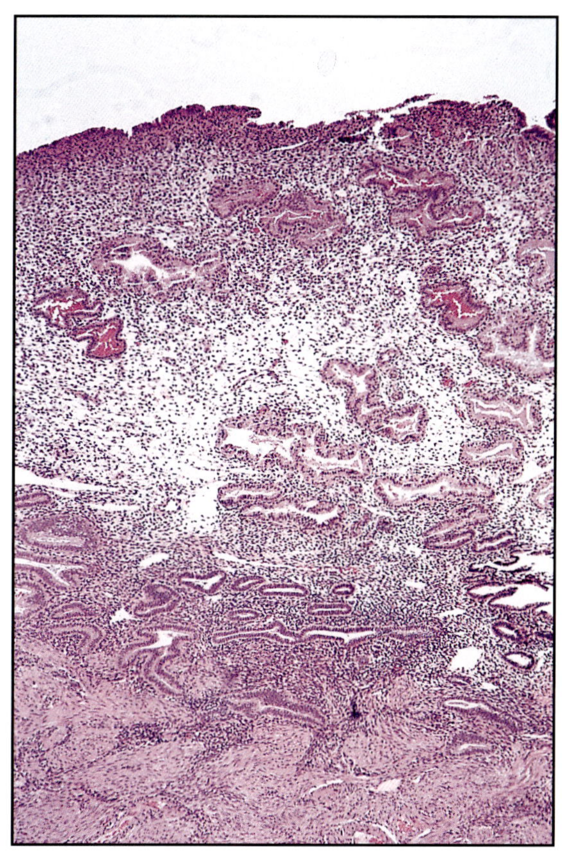

Image 2.2
Functionalis and basalis of the endometrium (secretory phase). The functionalis is fully responsive to hormonal stimulation and consists of secretory glands. The basalis is an inactive zone and consists of weakly proliferative glands and dense, spindled stroma. Histologic section (H&E, 100X).

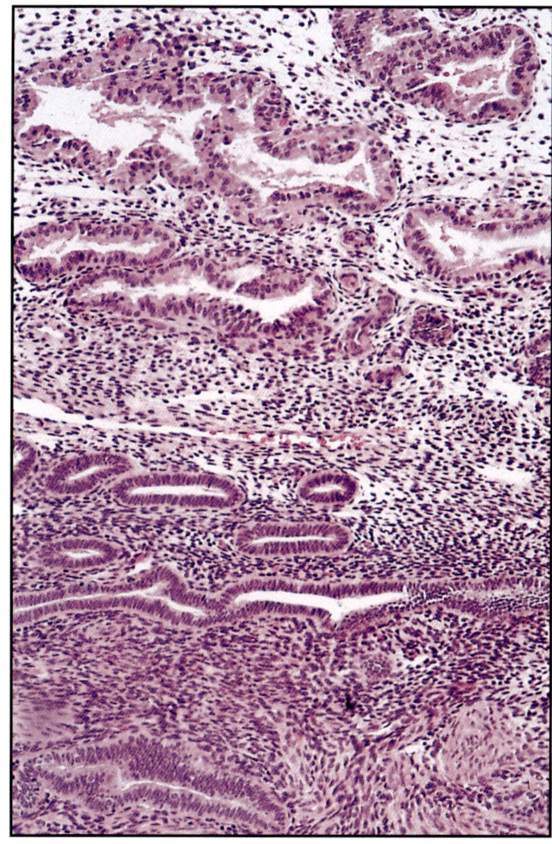

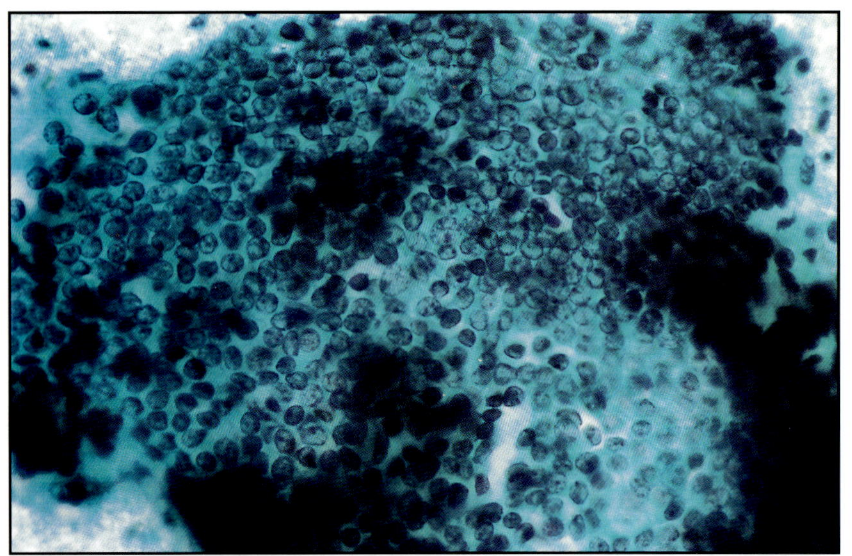

Image 2.3
Proliferative glandular cells of the endometrium. The proliferative glandular cells have scant cytoplasm and small ovoid nuclei with dense chromatin and inconspicuous nucleoli. They are arranged in a flat sheet with apparent nuclear crowding and overlapping. Endometrial brushing (Papanicolaou, 400X).

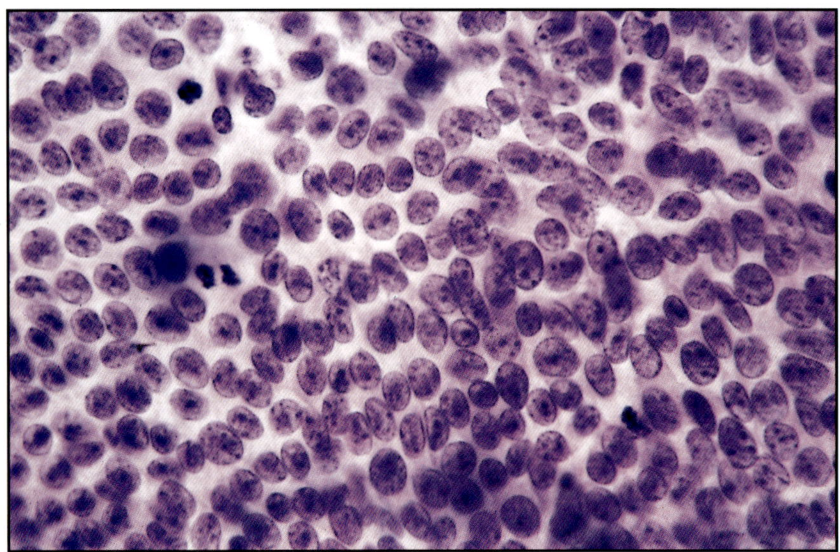

Image 2.4
Proliferative glandular cells of the endometrium. A flat sheet of proliferative glandular cells contains uniform and regular, ovoid nuclei with inconspicuous nucleoli. Note that mitotic figures are present. Endometrial brushing (Papanicolaou, 800X).

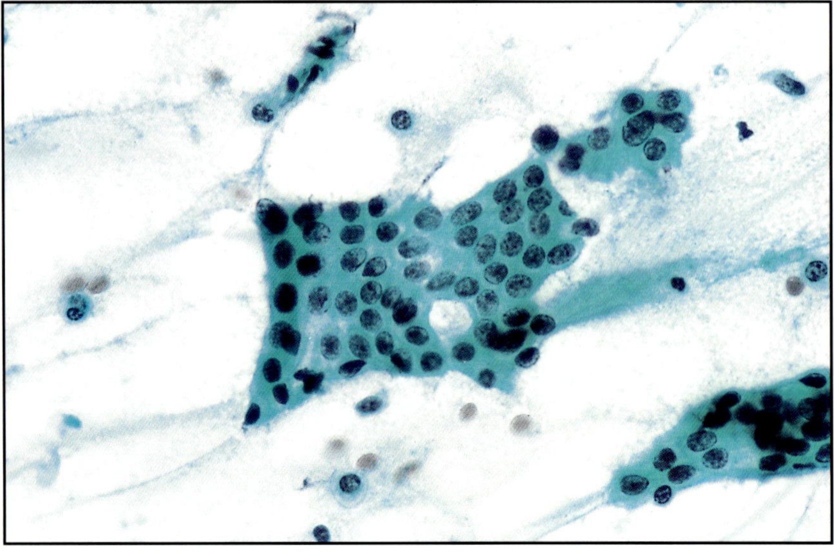

Image 2.5
Secretory glandular cells of the endometrium (ovulatory phase). The glandular cells have small, round or ovoid nuclei with dense chromatin and an increased amount of cytoplasm. Some of the glandular cells with partially perinuclear clearing intermingle with glandular cells with dense cytoplasm. Endometrial brushing (Papanicolaou, 400X).

Image 2.6
Secretory glandular cells of the endometrium (early secretory phase). The secretory glandular cells have clear cytoplasm and small ovoid nuclei with dense chromatin and inconspicuous nucleoli. They occur in sheet arrangements with a honeycomb pattern. Endometrial brushing (Papanicolaou, 400X).

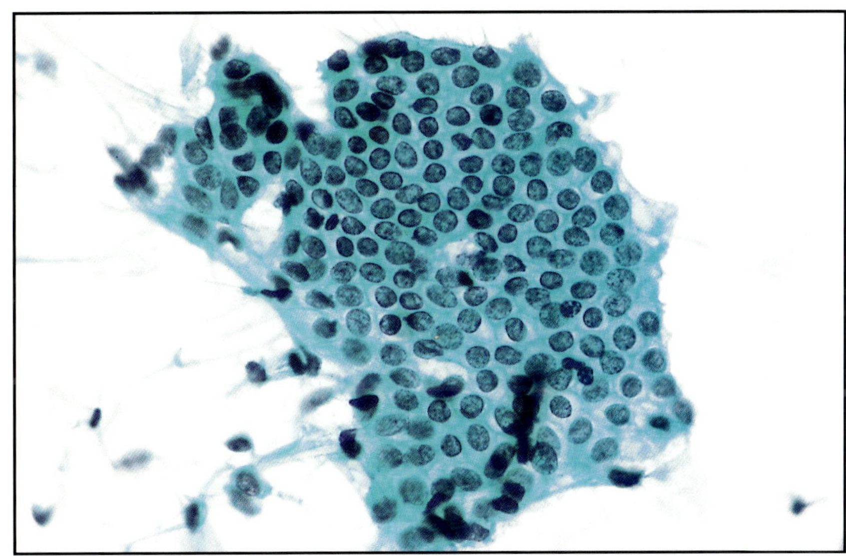

Image 2.7
Secretory glandular cells of the endometrium (midsecretory phase). The secretory glandular cells have a moderate amount of well-demarcated, clear cytoplasm and enlarged, round or slightly ovoid, vesicular nuclei with uniformly dispersed chromatin and occasional conspicuous nucleoli. They occur in a sheet arrangement with a honeycomb pattern. Endometrial brushing (Papanicolaou, 400X).

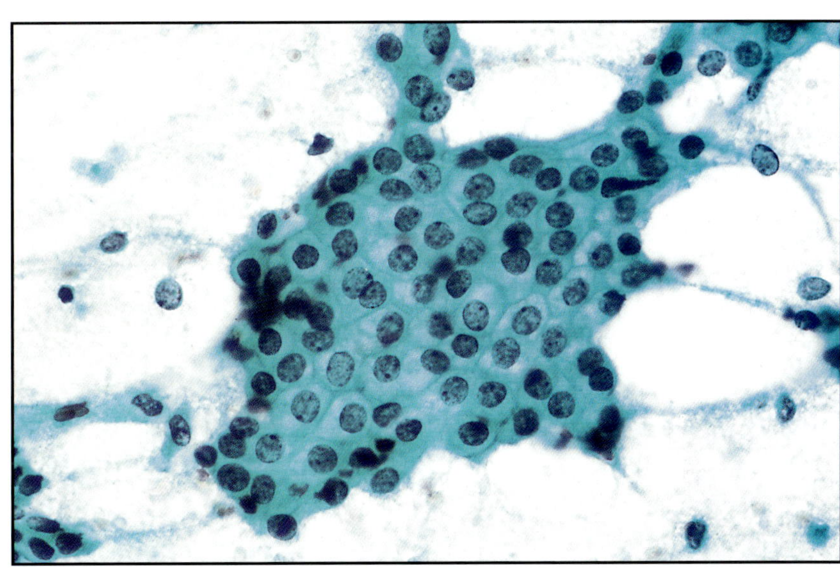

Image 2.8
Secretory glandular cells of the endometrium (late secretory phase). The secretory glandular cells have a moderate amount of well-demarcated, somewhat dense cytoplasm and round or ovoid nuclei with coarse chromatin. They occur in a sheet arrangement. Endometrial brushing (Papanicolaou, 400X).

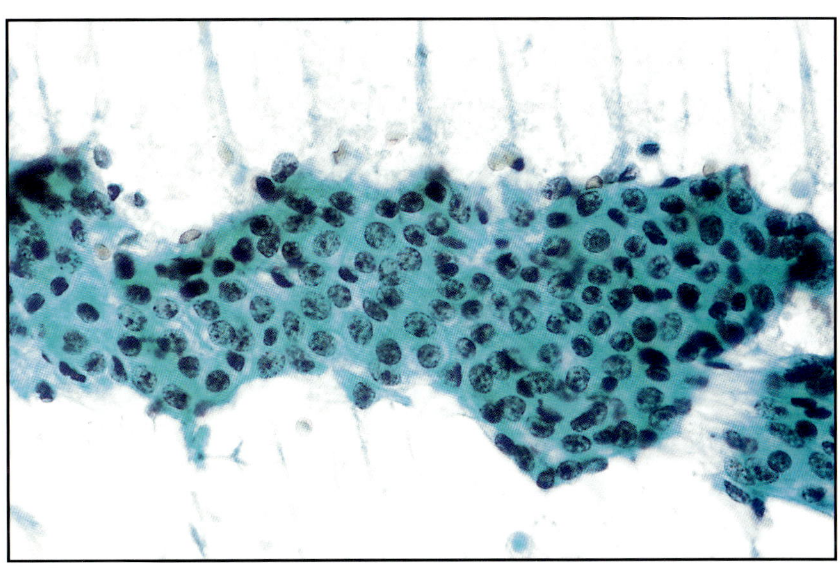

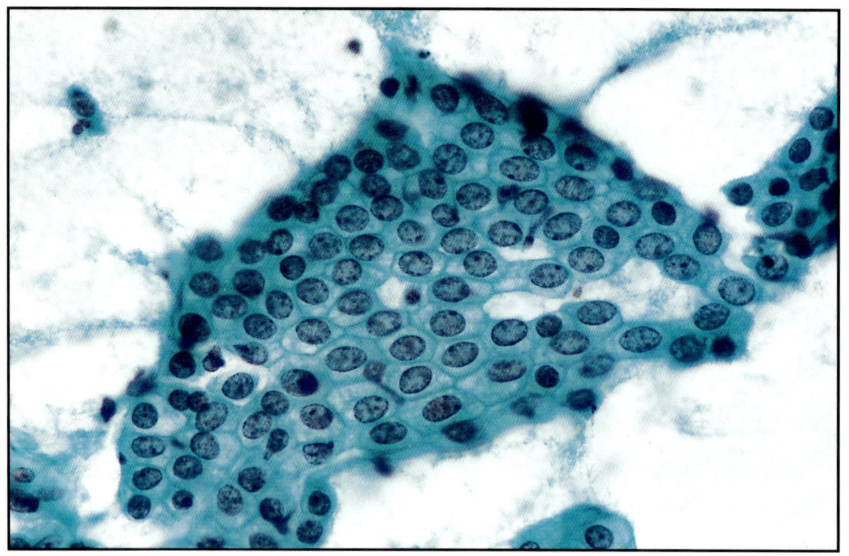

Image 2.9
Secretory glandular cells of the endometrium (early pregnancy). The glandular cells become "exaggerated" secretory cells and are enlarged. They have large, round or ovoid, vesicular nuclei and an abundance of well-demarcated, clear cytoplasm. They occur in a sheet arrangement with a honeycomb pattern. Endometrial brushing (Papanicolaou, 400X).

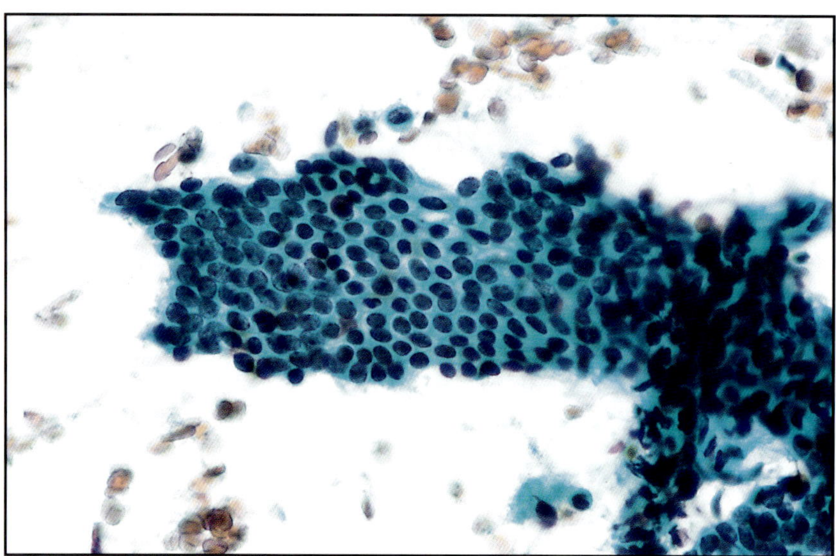

Image 2.10
Glandular cells of the atrophic endometrium. The glandular cells have small, round or ovoid, dense or pyknotic nuclei and scant, nonvacuolated cytoplasm. They occur in a sheet arrangement. Endometrial brushing (Papanicolaou, 400X).

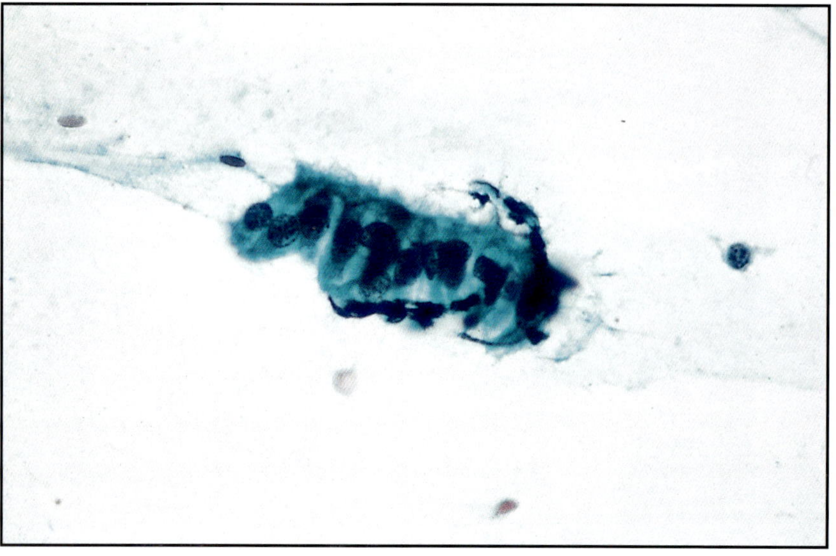

Image 2.11
Ciliated glandular cells of the endometrium. The glandular cells have well-developed cilia over their free margins and have centrally placed, ovoid vesicular nuclei with finely stippled chromatin. They are columnar in shape and arranged in a palisading fashion. Endometrial brushing (Papanicolaou, 400X).

Image 2.12
Ciliated glandular epithelium of the endometrium. The surface epithelium consists of ciliated columnar glandular cells with central, ovoid or elongated nuclei and brightly eosinophilic cytoplasm in a palisading arrangement (see Image 2.11). Histologic section (H&E, 200X).

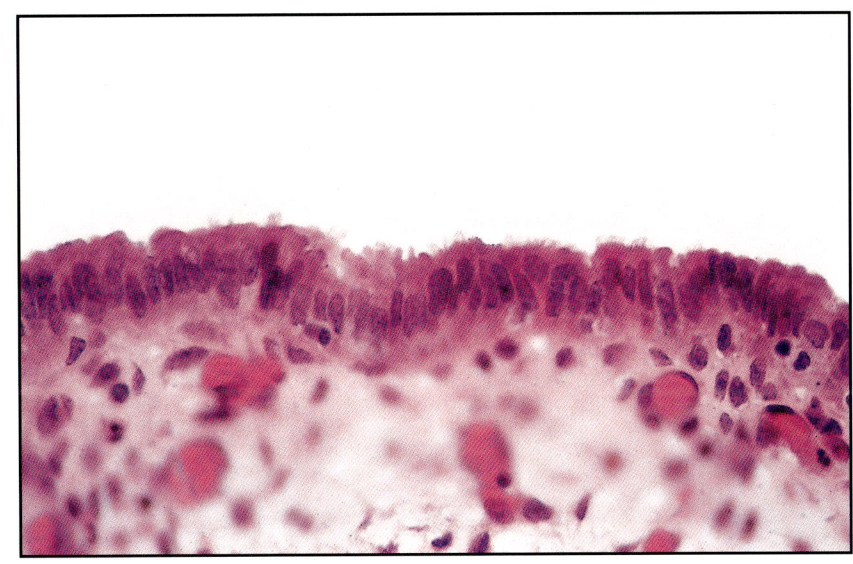

Image 2.13
Stromal cells of the endometrium (early proliferative phase). The stromal cells have scant, ill-defined cytoplasm and ovoid or fusiform nuclei with fine chromatin. They occur in loose, non-cohesive groupings. Endometrial brushing (Papanicolaou, 400X).

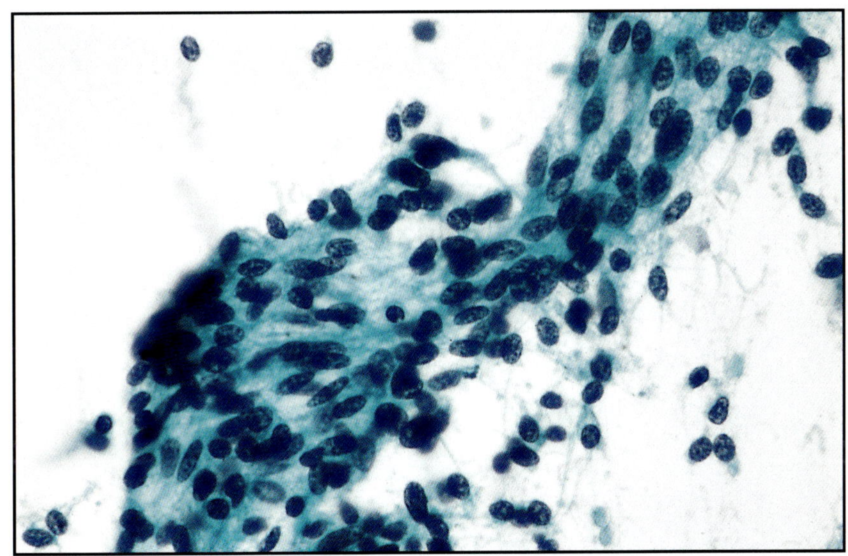

Image 2.14
Stromal cells of the endometrium (late proliferative phase). The stromal cells have a moderate amount to an abundance of ill-defined cytoplasm and ovoid or fusiform nuclei with somewhat dense chromatin. They occur in cohesive groupings. Endometrial brushing (Papanicolaou, 400X).

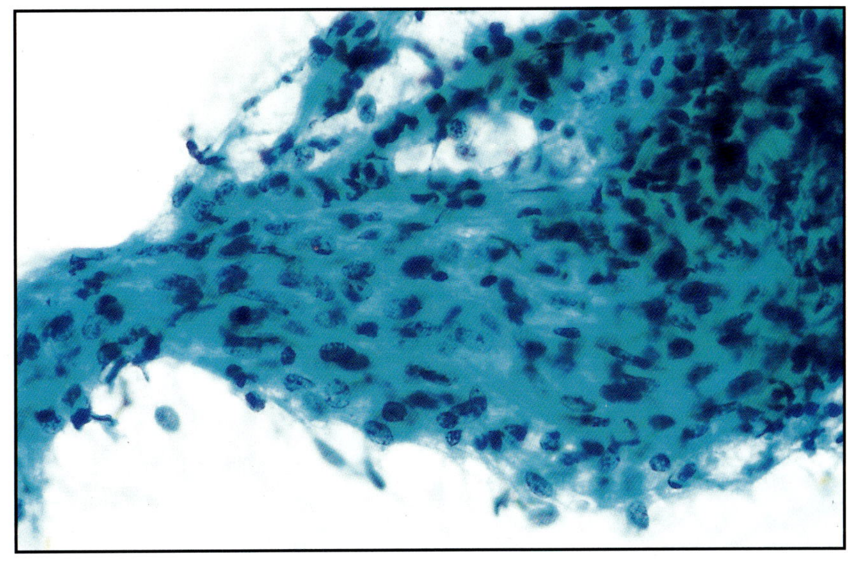

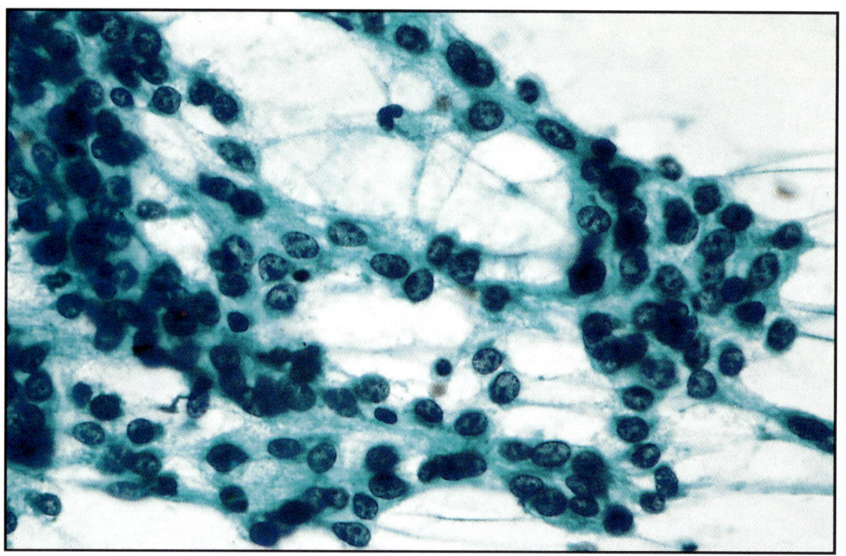

Image 2.15
Stromal cells of the endometrium (midsecretory phase). The stromal cells have scant, ill-defined cytoplasm and enlarged, plump, vesicular nuclei. They occur in loose, noncohesive groupings. Endometrial brushing (Papanicolaou, 400X).

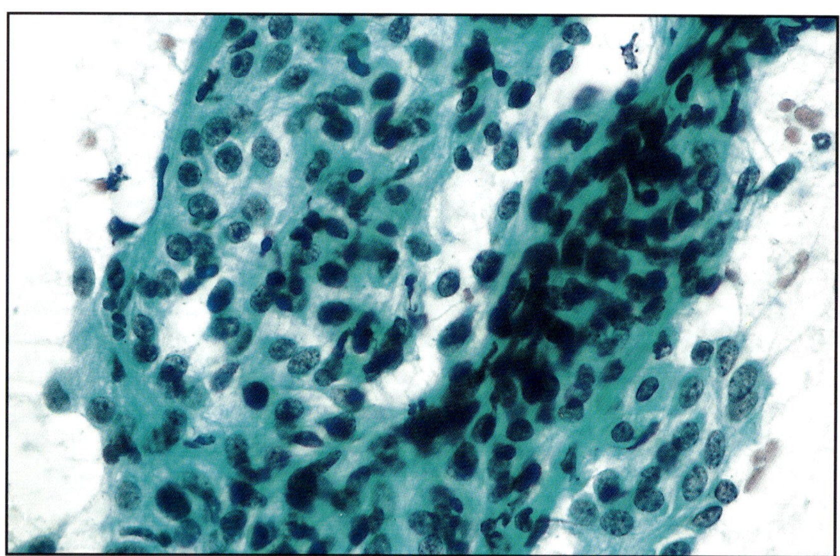

Image 2.16
Stromal cells of the endometrium (late secretory phase). The stromal cells in the upper portion of the endometrium undergo predecidual changes. They acquire more granular or dense cytoplasm and enlarged, ovoid nuclei, and occur in a loose or cohesive grouping. Endometrial brushing (Papanicolaou, 400X).

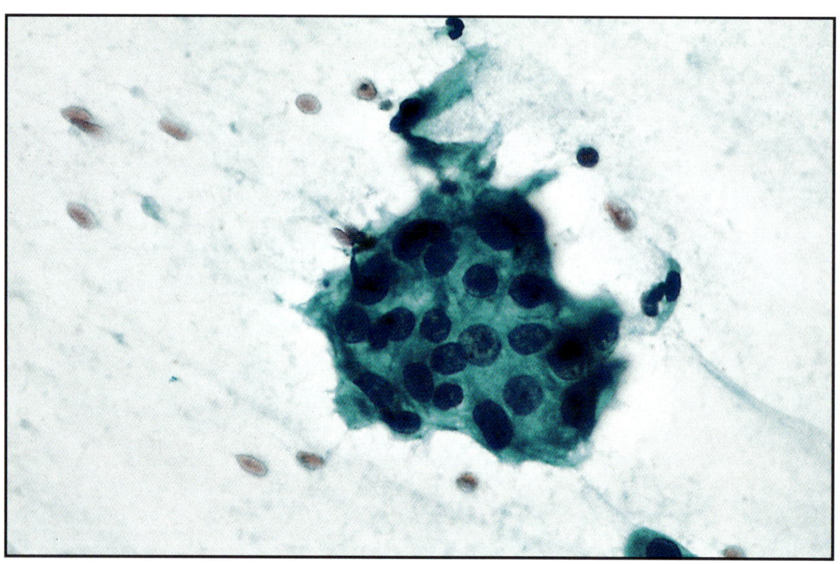

Image 2.17
Predecidual cells of the endometrium (late secretory phase). The predecidual cells (the predecidualized stromal cells) become increasingly enlarged. They have more abundant granular or dense cytoplasm and large ovoid nuclei, and occur in a cohesive grouping. Endometrial brushing (Papanicolaou, 400X).

Image 2.18
Predecidual cells of the endometrium
(late secretory phase). The predecidual
cells have an abundance of relatively
well-defined, dense cytoplasm and
large ovoid nuclei. They occur in sheet
arrangements. Note that nuclei exhibit
variation in nuclear size. Endometrial
brushing (Papanicolaou, 400X).

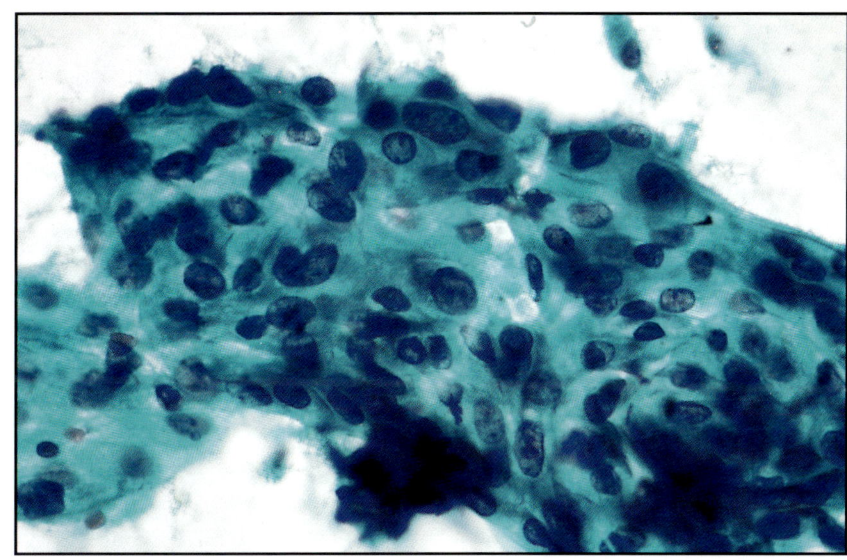

Image 2.19
Predecidual cells of the endometrium
(late secretory phase). Toward the end
of the late secretory phase, some of the
perivascular predecidual cells reach
very large size, resembling decidual
cells seen during pregnancy. They have
large vesicular nuclei with frequent
small or prominent nucleoli and well-
defined, dense cytoplasm, and occur in
a sheet arrangement. Endometrial
brushing (Papanicolaou, 400X).

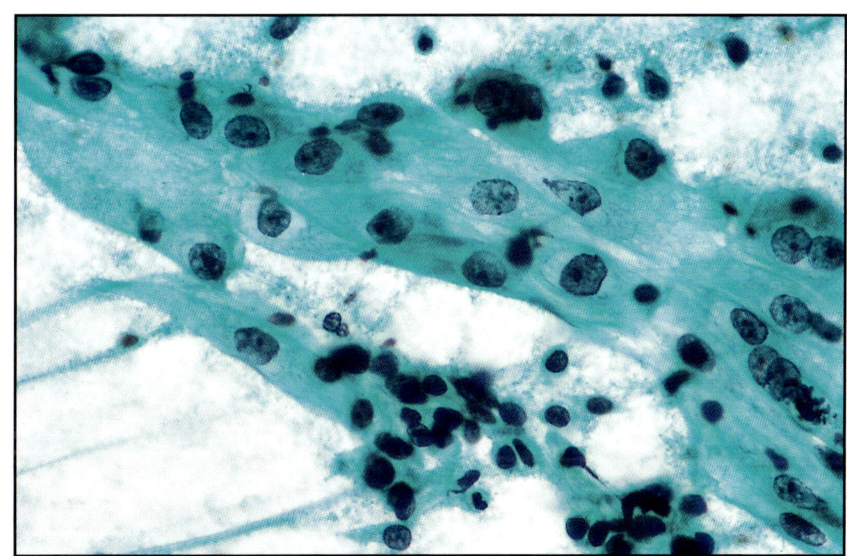

Image 2.20
Predecidual cells of the endometrium
(late secretory phase). At the end of the
late secretory phase, as the stroma begins
to disintegrate, many predecidual cells in
the upper portion of the endometrium
separate from each other and become
rounded. They have centrally placed,
round or ovoid nuclei and a moderate
amount of well-defined, finely granular
or dense cytoplasm, and occur in a
loose grouping. Endometrial brushing
(Papanicolaou, 400X).

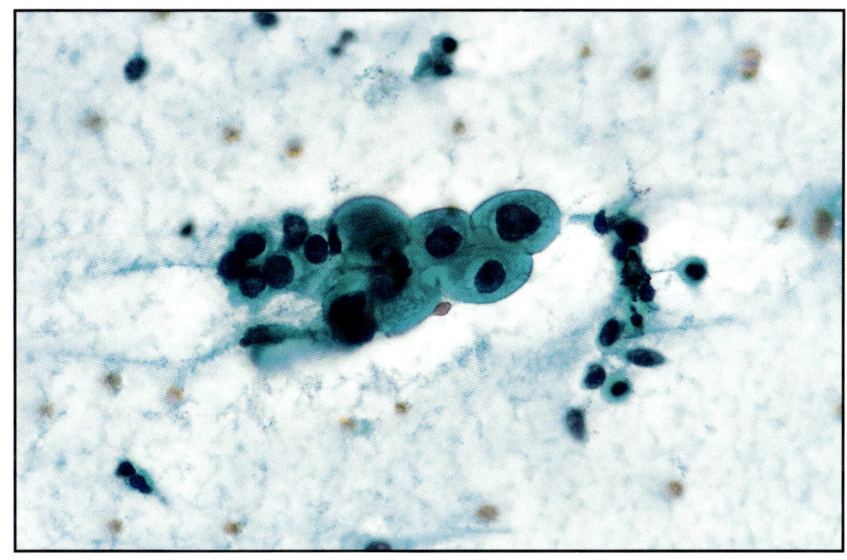

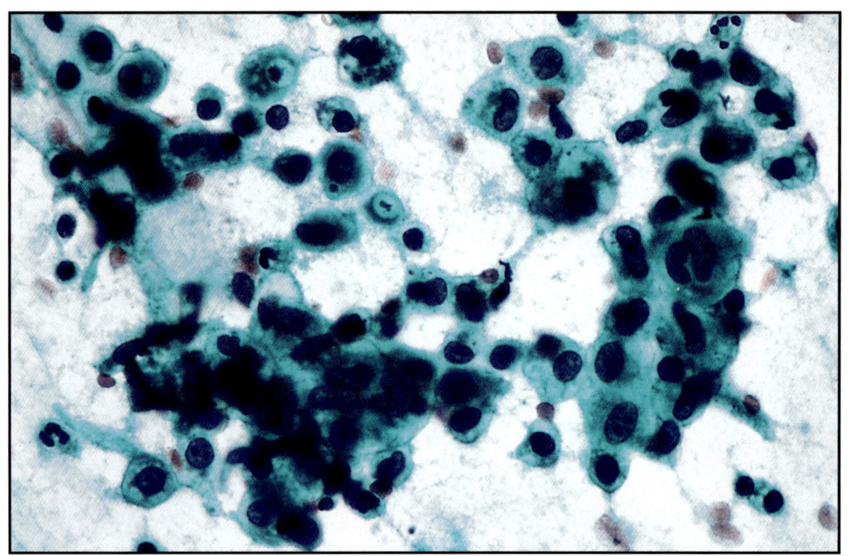

Image 2.21
Solitary predecidual cells of the endometrium (late secretory phase). At the end of the secretory phase, the predecidual cells separate from each other and occur in loose groupings or as solitary cells. They have round, ovoid, or bean-shaped nuclei and various amounts of relatively well-defined, foamy or finely granular cytoplasm, morphologically mimicking histiocytes. Cytoplasmic vacuoles are noticed, some of which contain neutrophils. Endometrial brushing (Papanicolaou, 400X).

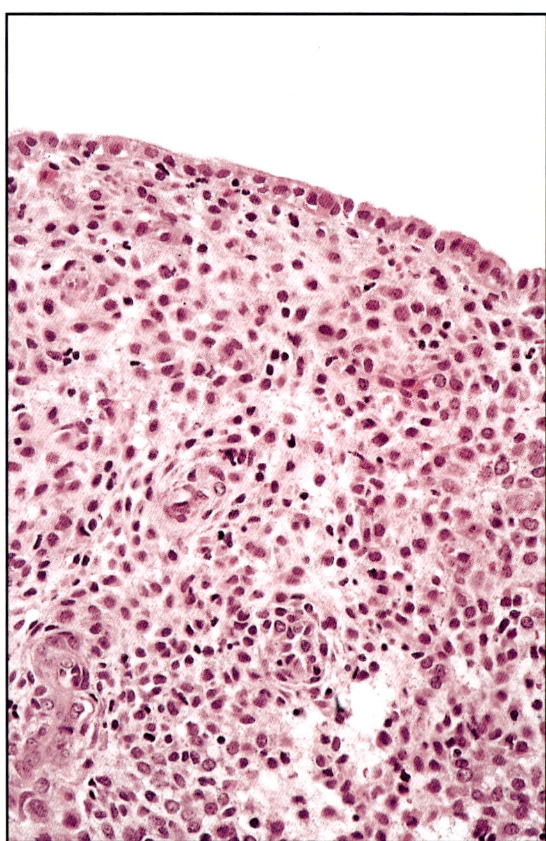

Image 2.22
Predecidualization of the endometrium (late secretory phase). The stromal cells undergo predecidual changes. Cuffs or islands of large predecidual cells are present around spiral arteries near the surface of the endometrium. Histologic section (H&E, 200X).

Image 2.23
Solitary predecidual cells of the endometrium (menstrual phase). The solitary predecidual cells have round, ovoid, or bean-shaped nuclei and various amounts of relatively well-defined, foamy or finely granular cytoplasm, morphologically mimicking histiocytes. During menstruation these cells appear in the endometrial cavity in large numbers and may also be seen as an exodus of histiocyte-like cells in cervicovaginal smears procured during or shortly after the menstrual phase. Endometrial brushing (Papanicolaou, 400X).

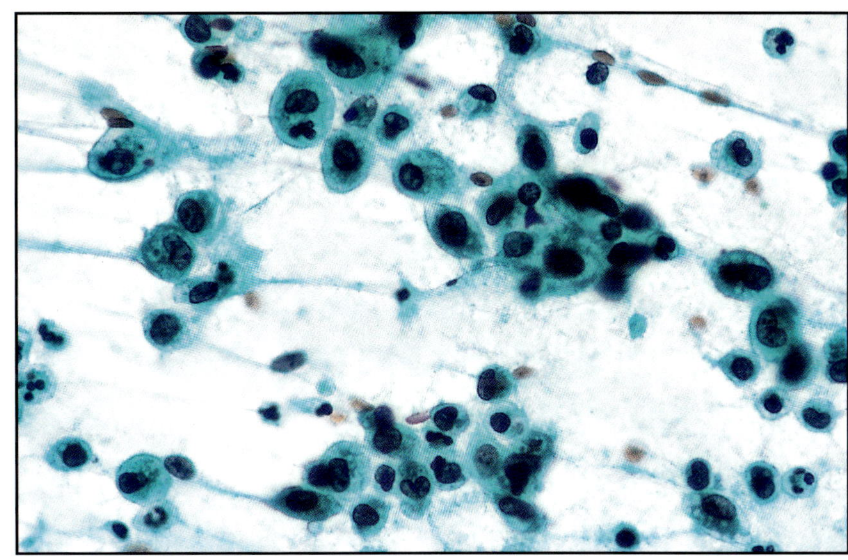

Image 2.24
Decidual cells of the endometrium (early pregnancy). The predecidual cells are converted to decidual cells during early pregnancy. These enlarged decidualized stromal cells have large vesicular nuclei and an abundance of well-defined, clear or foamy cytoplasm, and occur in a sheet arrangement. Endometrial brushing (Papanicolaou, 400X).

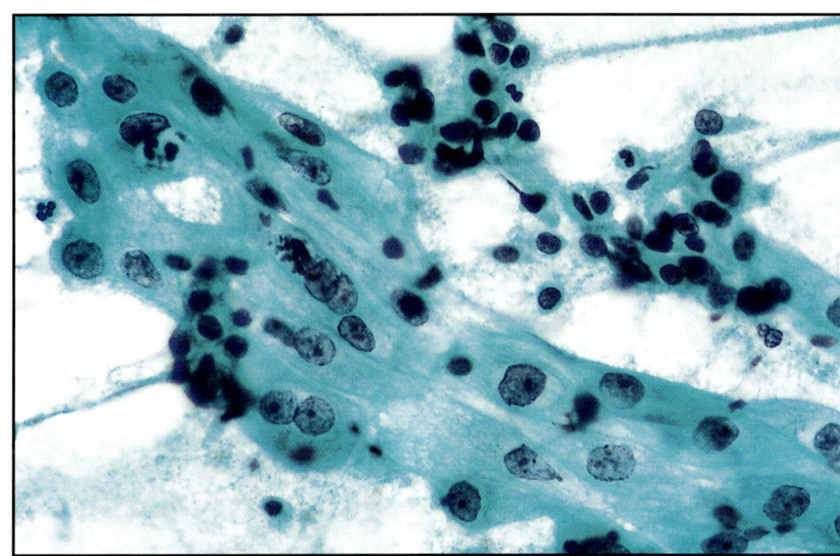

Image 2.25
Stromal cells of the atrophic endometrium. The stromal cells are spindled and closely packed. They have scant, ill-defined cytoplasm and plump, fusiform, or pyknotic nuclei, and occur in loose groupings. Endometrial brushing (Papanicolaou, 400X).

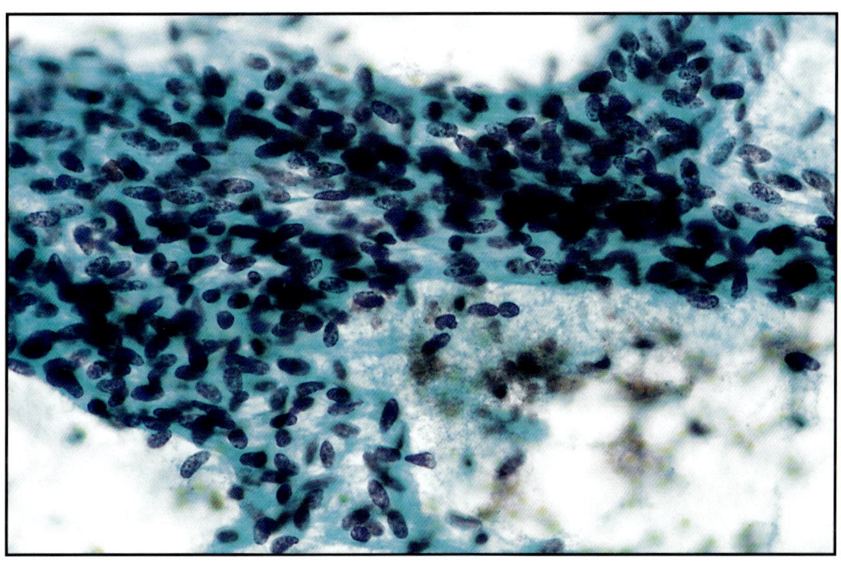

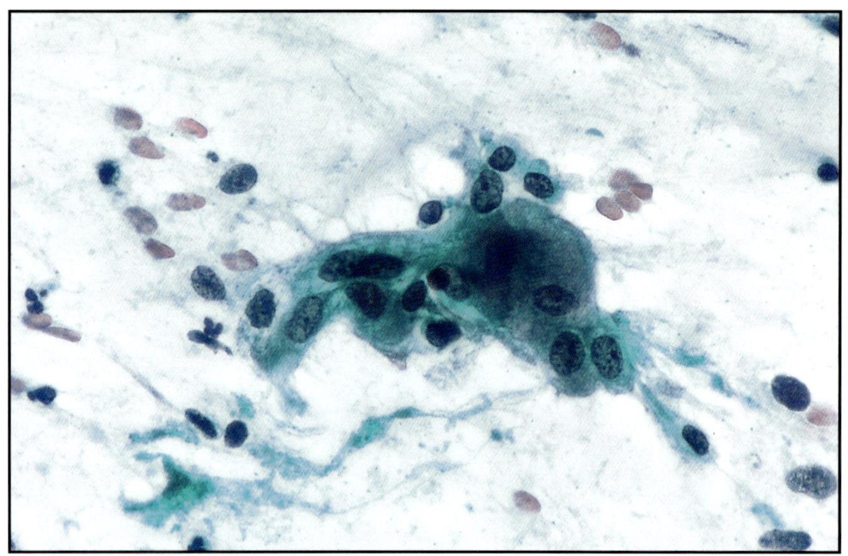

Image 2.26
Stromal foam cells in endometrial adenocarcinoma. The stromal foam cells have relatively large, centrally placed, ovoid nuclei with small nucleoli and a fine chromatin pattern, and an abundance of relatively well-defined, foamy cytoplasm. They occur in a three-dimensional, cohesive grouping. Endometrial brushing (Papanicolaou, 400X).

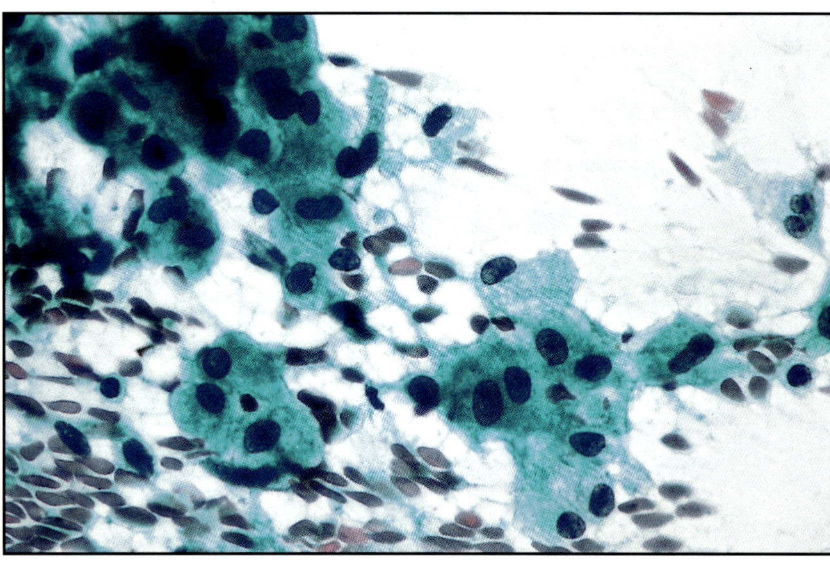

Image 2.27
Stromal foam cells in endometrial adenocarcinoma. The stromal foam cells have relatively large nuclei and an abundance of foamy cytoplasm, and occur in cohesive groupings. They are relatively uniform in size. These features distinguish them from morphologically similar foamy histiocytes that virtually always occur singly and are variable in size (see Image 2.33). Endometrial brushing (Papanicolaou, 400X).

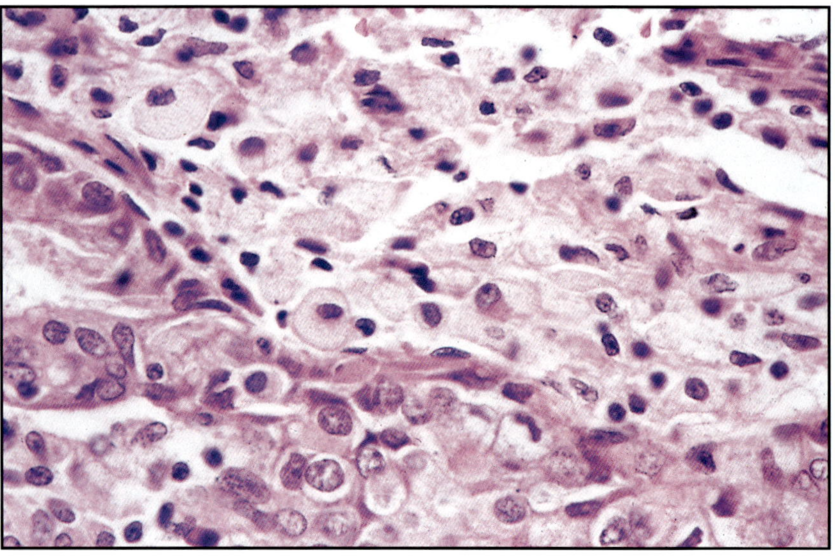

Image 2.28
Stromal foam cells in endometrial adenocarcinoma. Clusters of stromal foam cells with ovoid nuclei and an abundance of foamy cytoplasm (similar to those seen in Images 2.26 and 2.27) are present in the stroma of an endometrial adenocarcinoma. Histologic section (H&E, 200X).

Image 2.29

Stromal foam cells in endometrial adenocarcinoma. Groups of stromal foam cells with an abundance of foamy cytoplasm admix with some transitional-type cells with less abundant, finely granular cytoplasm, morphologically between stromal foam cells and regular stromal cells. Endometrial brushing (Papanicolaou, 400X).

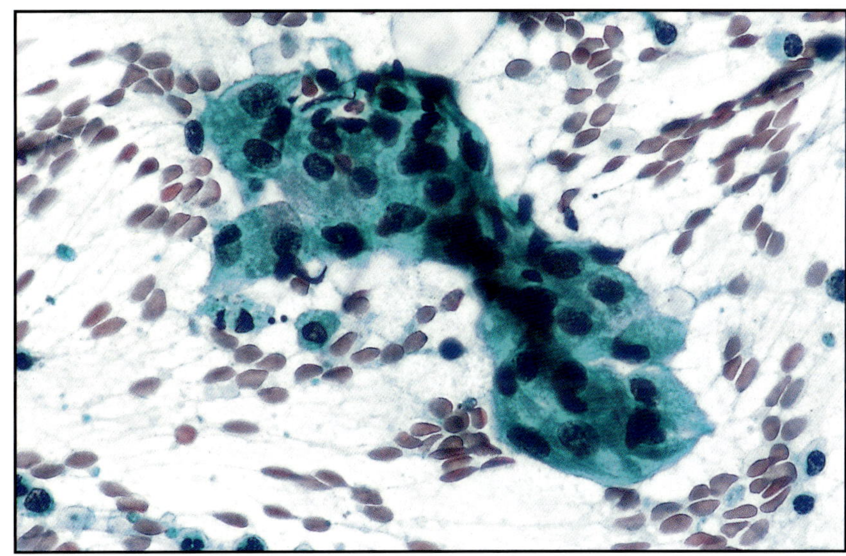

Image 2.30

Stromal foam cells in endometrial adenocarcinoma. Groups of typical stromal foam cells with an abundance of foamy cytoplasm (as shown in Image 2.27) next to clusters of transitional-type cells with less abundant, finely granular cytoplasm (as shown in Image 2.29) are present between glandular structures of an endometrial adenocarcinoma. Histologic section (H&E, 100X).

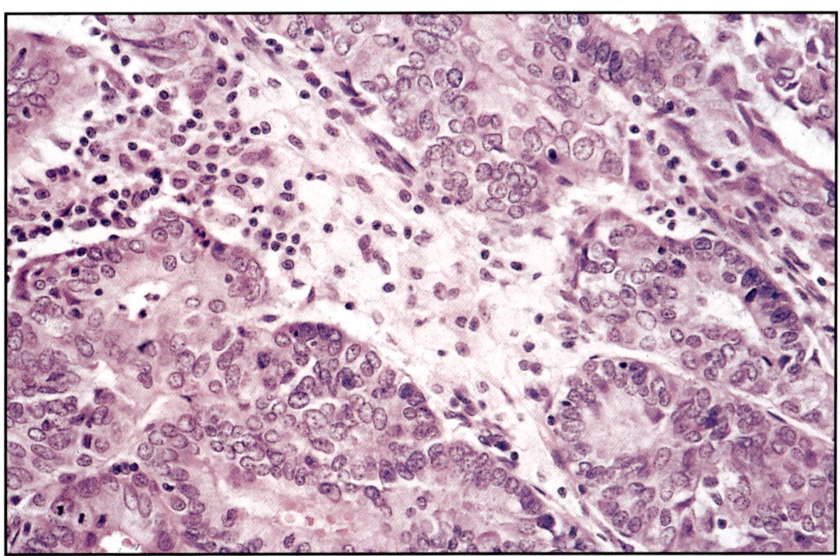

Image 2.31

Stromal foam cells in endometrial adenocarcinoma. Clusters of stromal foam cells have ovoid nuclei and an abundance of clear cytoplasm, and admix with stromal cells that have fusiform nuclei and ill-defined cytoplasm. The clear cytoplasm of stromal foam cells is rich in neutral fats. Endometrial brushing (Papanicolaou, 400X).

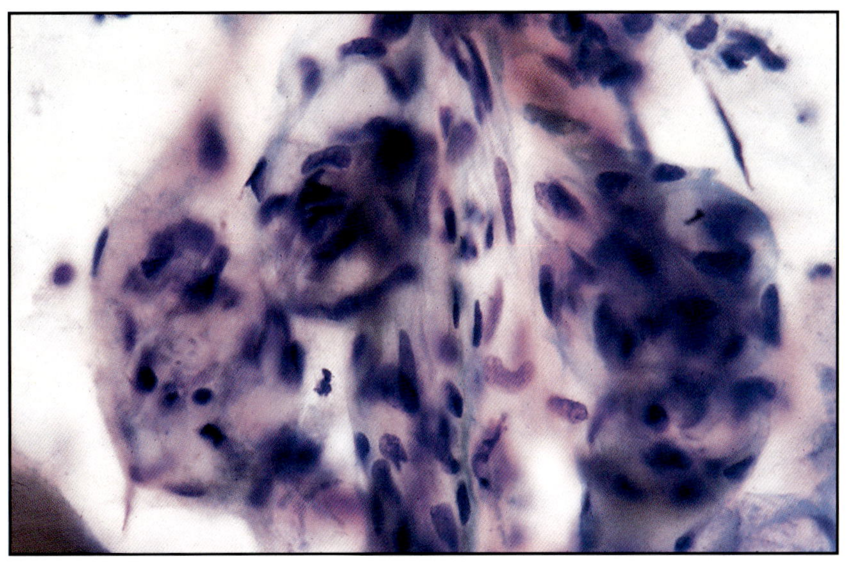

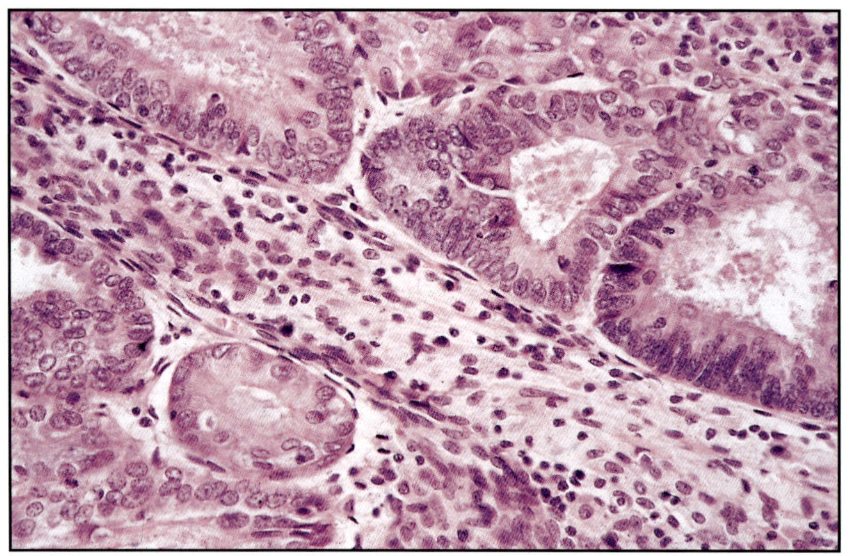

Image 2.32

Stromal foam cells in endometrial adenocarcinoma. A column of stromal foam cells with an abundance of clear cytoplasm (see Image 2.31) surrounded by stromal cells with fusiform nuclei and scant cytoplasm is present between glandular structures of an endometrial adenocarcinoma. Histologic section (H&E, 100X).

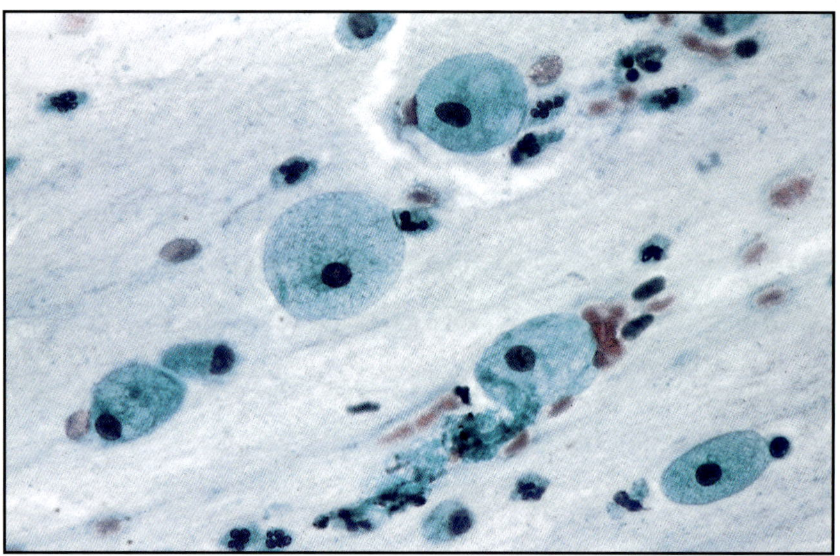

Image 2.33

Foamy histiocytes. The foamy histiocytes have relatively small, ovoid or bean-shaped, peripherally located nuclei and well-defined, foamy or vacuolated cytoplasm. They occur as solitary cells. Note that foamy histiocytes are variable in size (compare these cells with those shown in Images 2.26 and 2.27). Endometrial brushing (Papanicolaou, 400X).

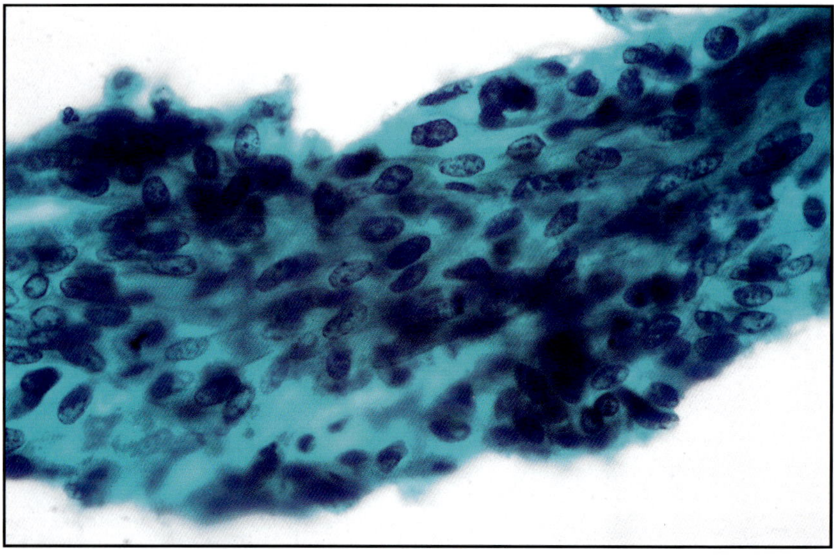

Image 2.34

Smooth muscle cells from the myometrium. The smooth muscle cells have ovoid or blunt-ended elongated nuclei with fine chromatin and an abundance of ill-defined cytoplasm, and occur in cohesive groupings. Note that the nuclei are in polar arrangements and the cells have ill-defined boundaries, giving a syncytial appearance (compare smooth muscle cells with predecidual cells shown in Image 2.18). Endometrial brushing (Papanicolaou, 400X).

Image 2.35
Smooth muscle of the myometrium.
Smooth muscle cells have ovoid, fusiform, or blunt-ended elongated nuclei
and abundant cytoplasmic matrix, and
are present in interlacing bundles.
Histologic section (H&E, 100X).

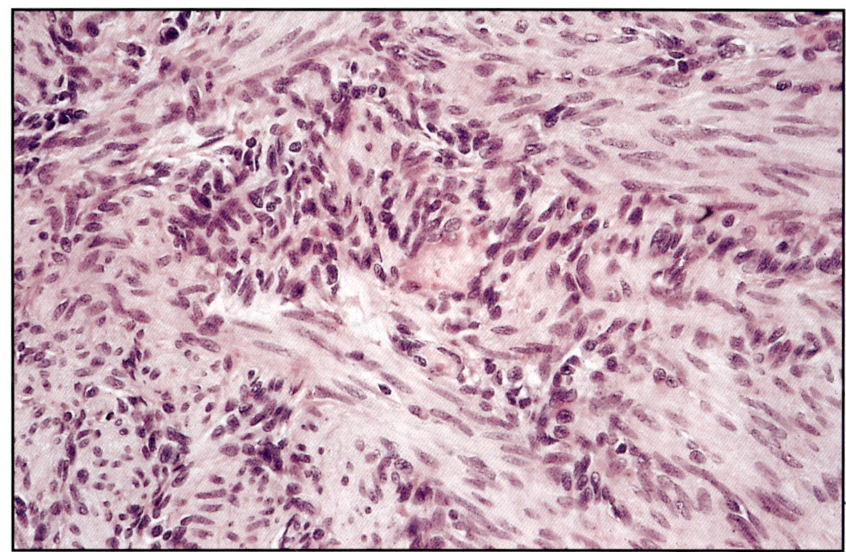

Image 2.36
Endometrium of the early proliferative
phase. Segments of straight, tubular
glands are composed of proliferative
glandular cells with scant cytoplasm.
Apparent nuclear crowding and overlapping are noted. The background is
relatively clean. Endometrial brushing
(Papanicolaou, 100X).

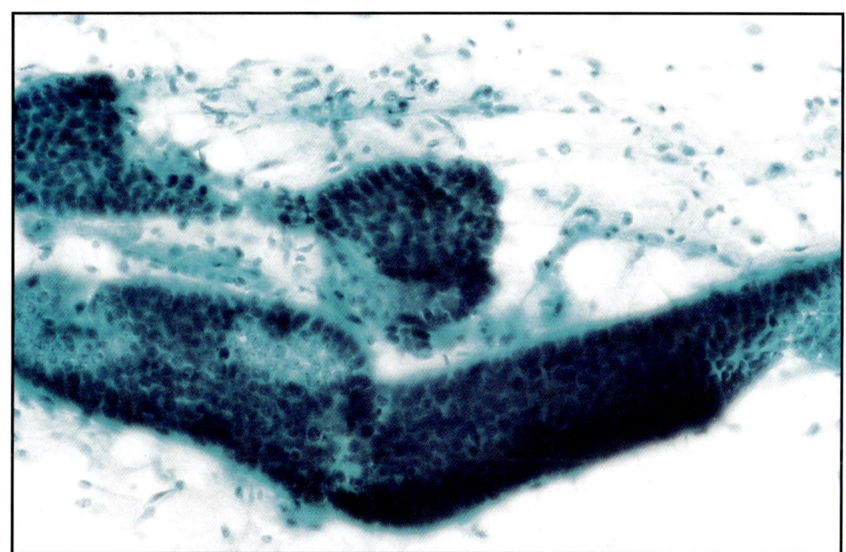

Image 2.37
Endometrium of the early proliferative
phase. The proliferative glandular cells
have scant cytoplasm and small, ovoid
nuclei with somewhat dense chromatin. They occur in cohesive, flat
sheet arrangements with nuclear
crowding and overlapping. Endometrial brushing (Papanicolaou, 400X).

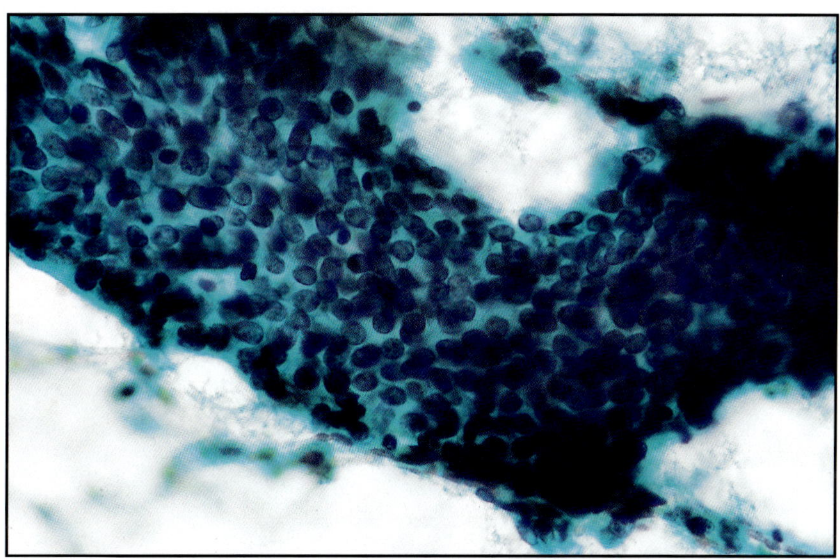

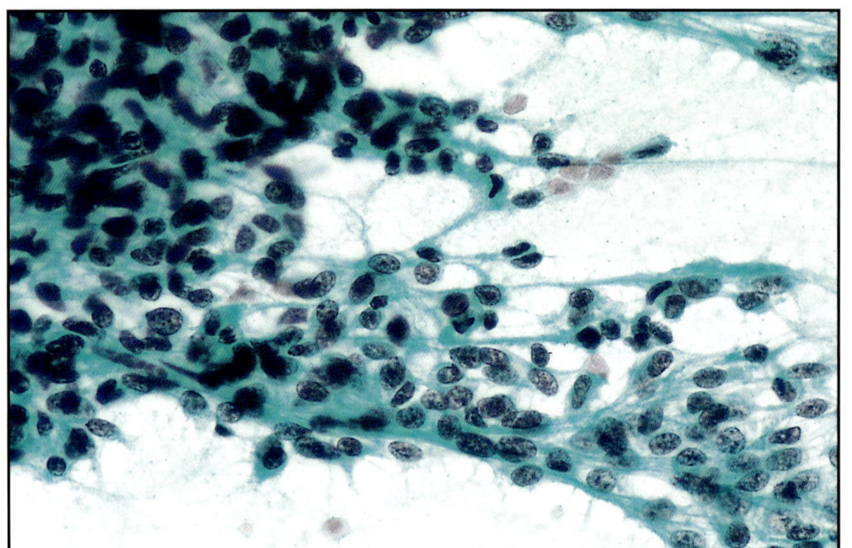

Image 2.38
Endometrium of the early proliferative phase. The stromal cells have scant, ill-defined cytoplasm and ovoid or fusiform nuclei with slightly dense chromatin and no recognizable nucleoli. They occur in loose, noncohesive groupings. Endometrial brushing (Papanicolaou, 400X).

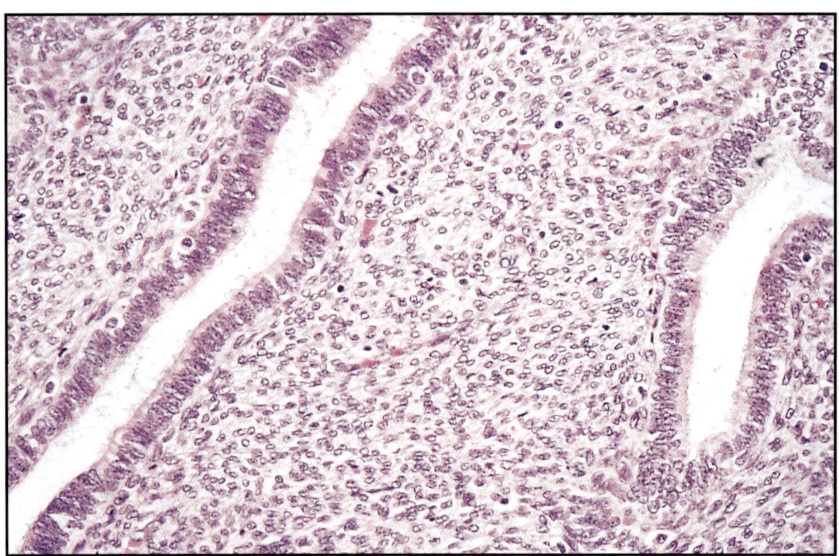

Image 2.39
Endometrium of the early proliferative phase. The glands are lined by pseudo-stratified columnar cells with high nuclear/cytoplasmic ratios and relatively dense chromatin. The glands are straight, have small diameter, and are dispersed in a relatively dense stroma. Histologic section (H&E, 200X).

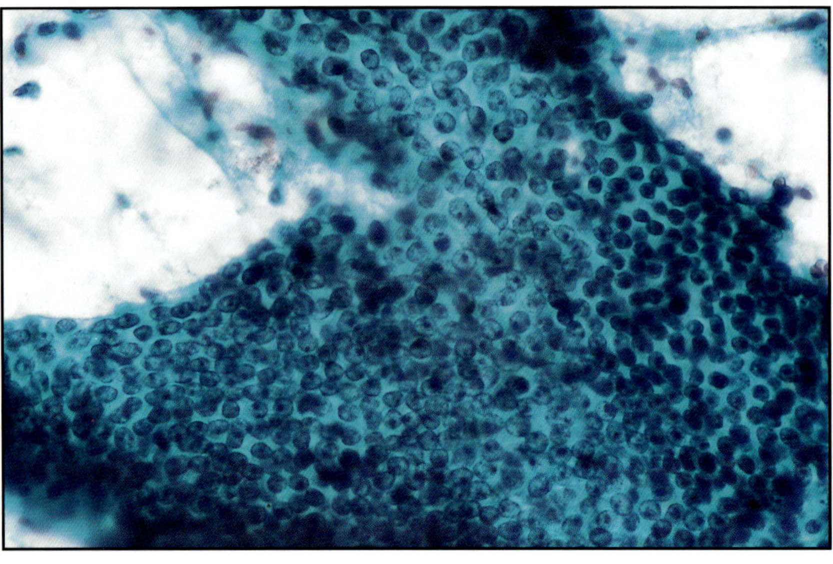

Image 2.40
Endometrium of the midproliferative phase. Flat sheets of proliferative glandular cells contain uniform and regular, round or ovoid nuclei with frequent small nucleoli and slightly dense chromatin. Nuclear crowding and overlapping are apparent. The cytologic features are similar to those shown in Image 2.37, except that there are no straight, tubular glands and the glandular cells show small nucleoli. Endometrial brushing (Papanicolaou, 400X).

Image 2.41

Endometrium of the midproliferative phase. The stromal cells acquire a moderate amount of ill-defined cytoplasm and ovoid or fusiform nuclei with slightly dense chromatin. They occur in loose or cohesive groupings. Endometrial brushing (Papanicolaou, 400X).

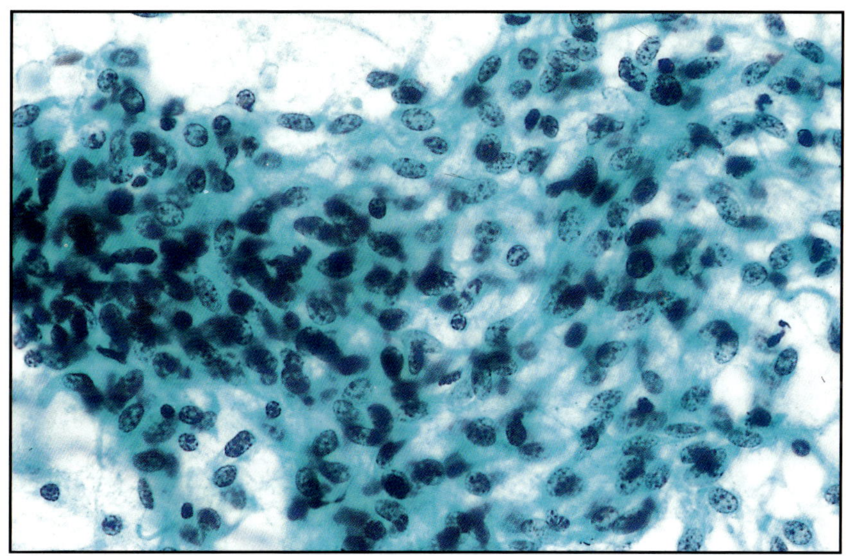

Image 2.42

Endometrium of the midproliferative phase. The glands have convoluted contours. The nuclei of proliferative glandular cells are ovoid or slightly elongated, have small nucleoli, and are found at the base of the cell. The stromal edema is present. Histologic section (H&E, 200X).

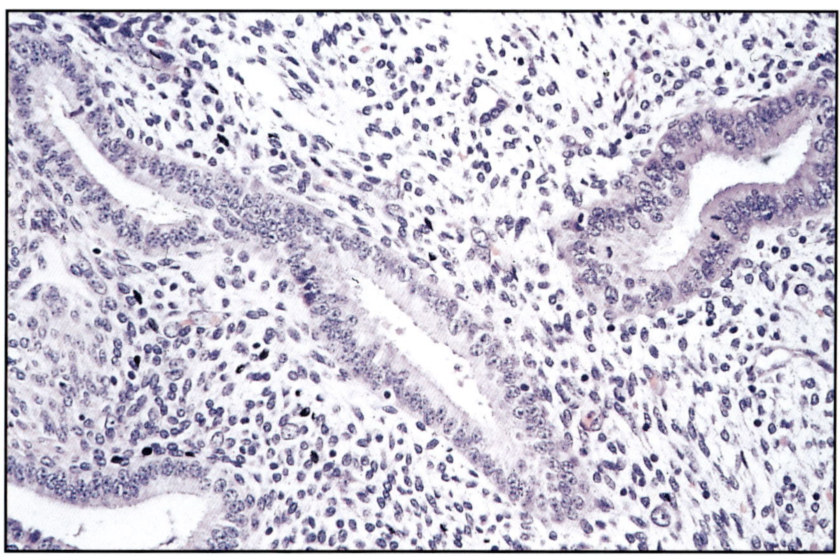

Image 2.43

Endometrium of the late proliferative phase. A low-power view of the endometrial cells exhibits crowding of the proliferative glandular cells with dense nuclei and abundant spindled stromal cells in cohesive groupings. Endometrial brushing (Papanicolaou, 100X).

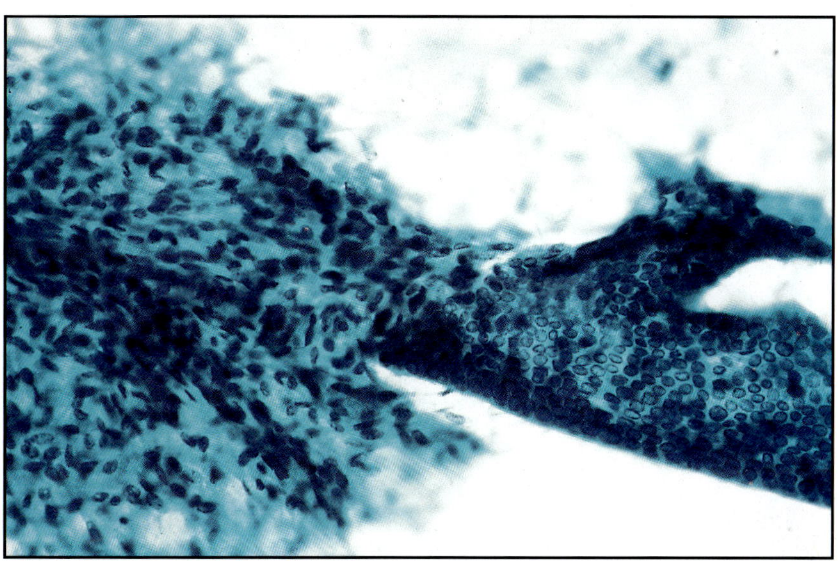

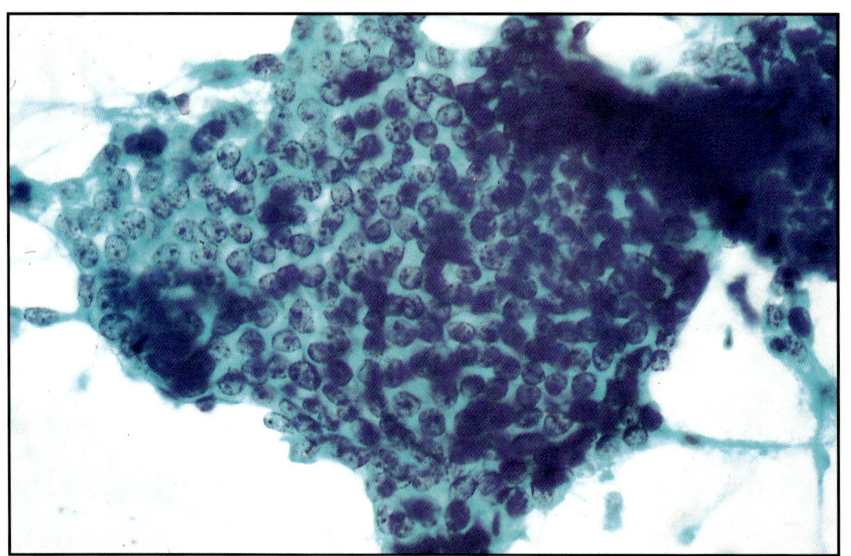

Image 2.44
Endometrium of the late proliferative phase. The proliferative glandular cells have uniform and regular, round or ovoid nuclei with frequent small nucleoli and scant cytoplasm. They occur in flat sheets with apparent nuclear crowding and overlapping. The cytologic features are identical to those shown in Image 2.40. Endometrial brushing (Papanicolaou, 400X).

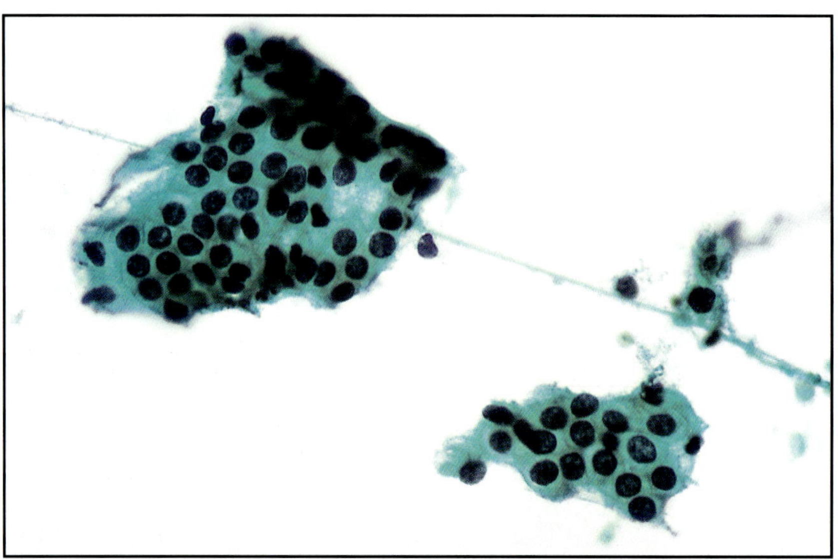

Image 2.45
Endometrium of the late proliferative phase. The glandular cells have small, dense nuclei and an increased amount of cytoplasm with scattered partially perinuclear clearing (corresponding to small subnuclear vacuoles seen on histologic sections). They occur in sheet arrangements without nuclear crowding and overlapping. This change (partially perinuclear clearing) is occasionally encountered toward the end of the late proliferative phase. Endometrial brushing (Papanicolaou, 400X).

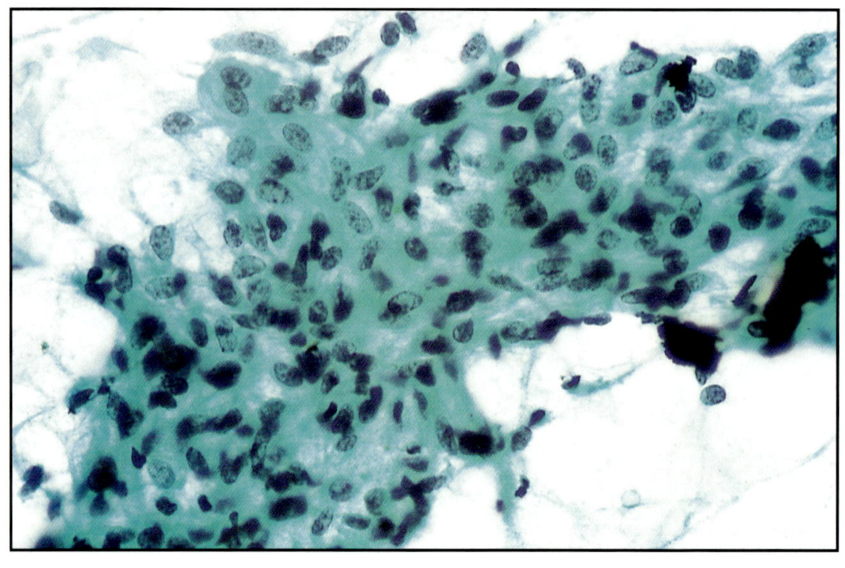

Image 2.46
Endometrium of the late proliferative phase. The stromal cells have an abundance of ill-defined cytoplasm and ovoid or fusiform nuclei with dense chromatin, and occur in cohesive groupings. They appear spindled and are similar to those shown in Image 2.41. Endometrial brushing (Papanicolaou, 400X).

Image 2.47
Endometrium of the late proliferative phase. The glands remain convoluted, as seen in the midproliferative phase. Their contours become more sinuous and their diameters increase as well. The nuclei of glandular cells are ovoid or slightly elongated and found at the base of the cell. Mitotic figures are noted. Histologic section (H&E, 200X).

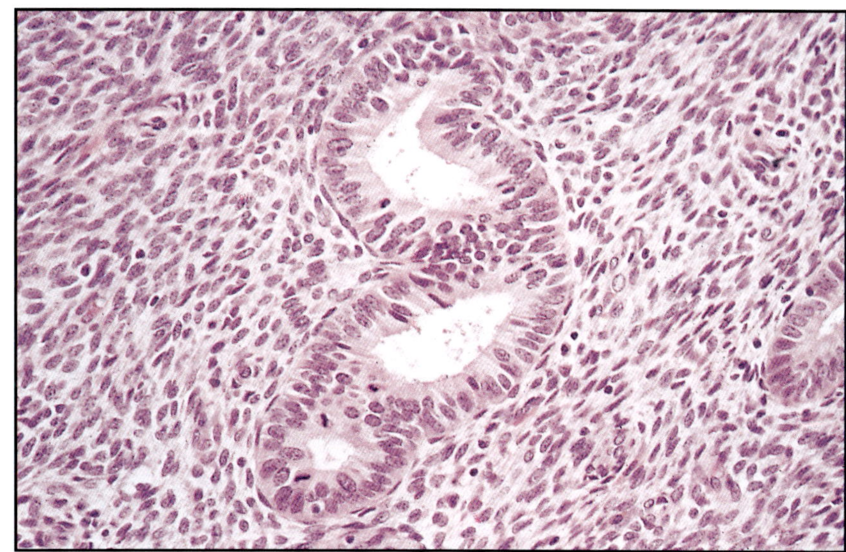

Image 2.48
Endometrium of the ovulatory phase. A low-power view of the endometrial cells exhibits a large sheet of proliferative glandular cells intermixed with a small sheet of secretory glandular cells. The findings are morphologically similar to those seen during the late proliferative phase, except that the proliferative glandular cells appear less crowded and there are more secretory glandular cells with partially clear cytoplasm. Endometrial brushing (Papanicolaou, 100X).

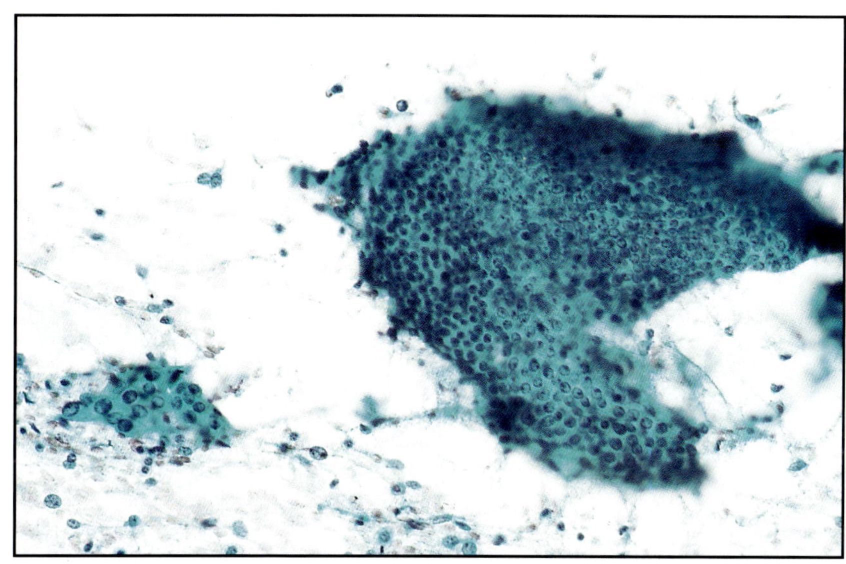

Image 2.49
Endometrium of the ovulatory phase. The secretory glandular cells have a small amount of clear or partially clear cytoplasm and relatively small, round or ovoid, dense nuclei. They occur in a sheet arrangement. Endometrial brushing (Papanicolaou, 400X).

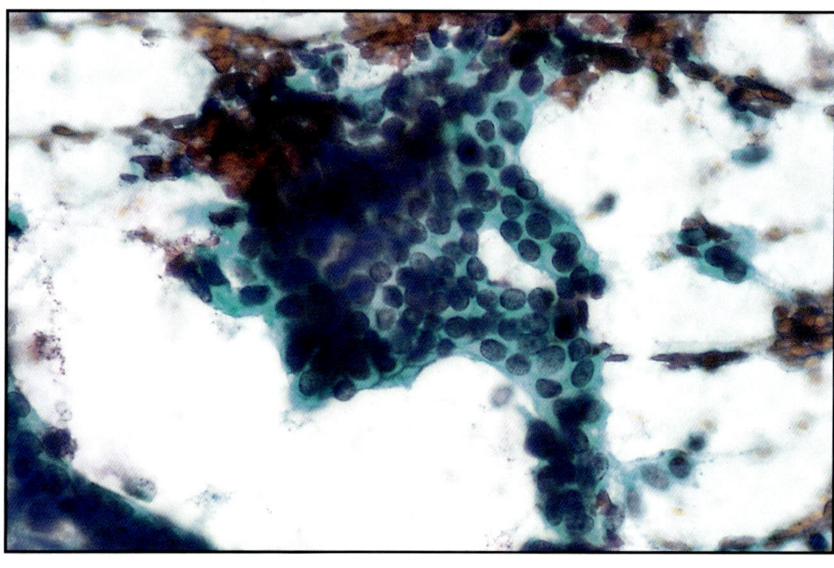

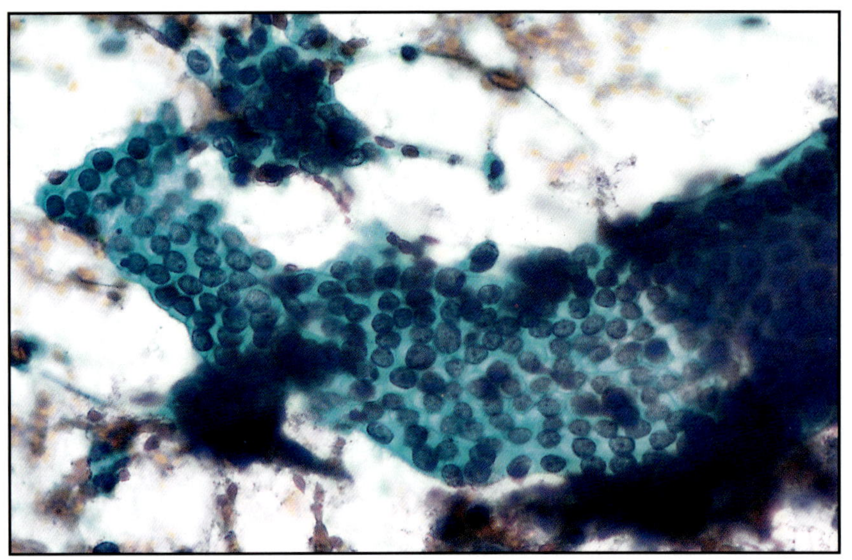

Image 2.50
Endometrium of the ovulatory phase. The secretory glandular cells have a small amount of well-defined, clear or partially clear cytoplasm (compare these cells with secretory glandular cells shown in Image 2.45), and occur in a monolayer sheet arrangement without nuclear crowding and overlapping. Note that the background is still clean. Endometrial brushing (Papanicolaou, 400X).

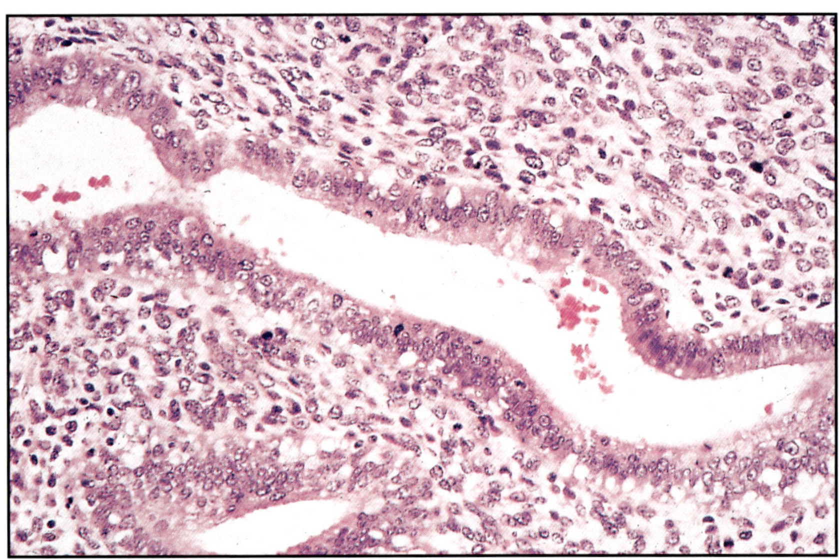

Image 2.51
Endometrium of the ovulatory phase. Some glandular cells have small subnuclear glycogen vacuoles, and many glandular cells are devoid of vacuoles. Nuclear pseudostratification is maintained. The overall histology is that of the late proliferative phase endometrium, except that there are more small subnuclear vacuoles. Histologic section (H&E, 200X).

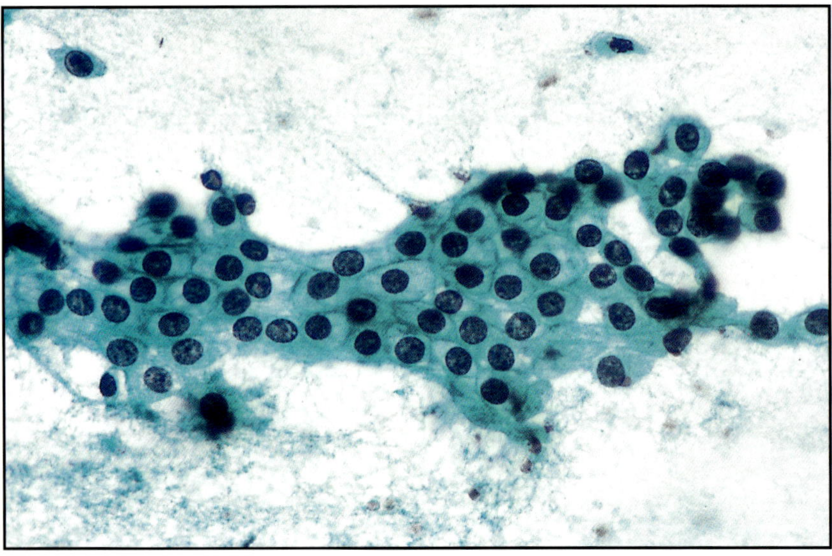

Image 2.52
Endometrium of the early secretory phase. The secretory glandular cells have an abundance of well-defined, clear or partially clear cytoplasm and larger, round or ovoid nuclei with dense chromatin. They occur in sheet arrangements with a honeycomb pattern. Note that the background is slightly mucoid. Endometrial brushing (Papanicolaou, 400X).

Image 2.53
Endometrium of the early secretory phase. Some of the secretory glandular cells with clear or partially clear cytoplasm intermix with glandular cells with relatively dense cytoplasm. This probably reflects that the distribution of glycogen contents among different glandular cells is uneven during this period. Endometrial brushing (Papanicolaou, 400X).

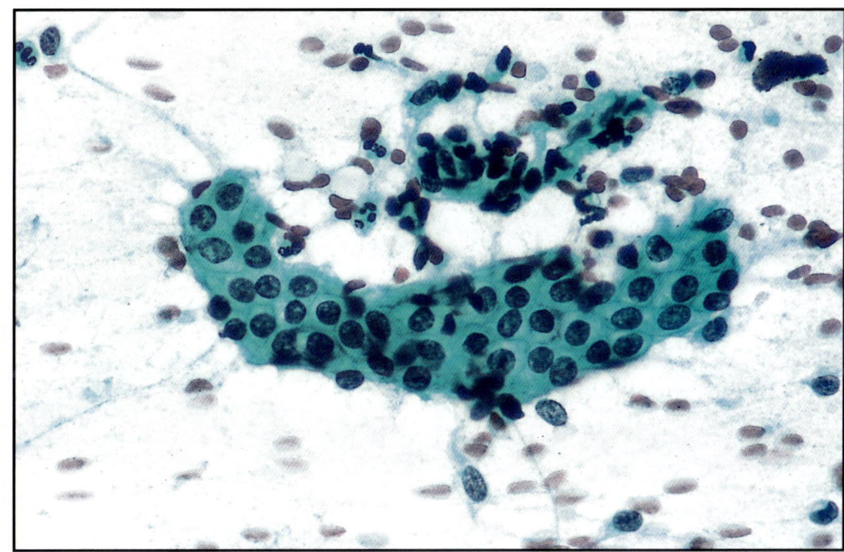

Image 2.54
Endometrium of the early secretory phase. The stromal cells have an abundance of ill-defined cytoplasm and ovoid or fusiform nuclei with dense chromatin, and occur in cohesive groupings. They appear spindled and have the same appearance as they had during the late proliferative phase. Endometrial brushing (Papanicolaou, 400X).

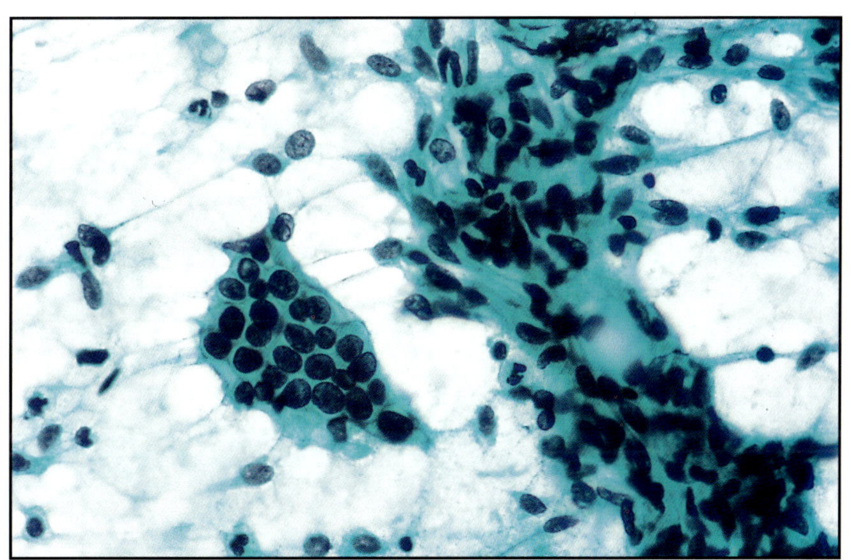

Image 2.55
Endometrium of the early secretory phase. Numerous glandular cells containing large, well-developed subnuclear vacuoles and exhibiting nuclear palisading are present—a finding typical of day 17. Stromal edema is noticed. The first unequivocal light microscopic indication that ovulation has occurred is the presence of subnuclear vacuoles involving more than 50% of the endometrial glands as in this case. During this phase, the vacuoles shift from a subnuclear to a supranuclear location. Histologic section (H&E, 200X).

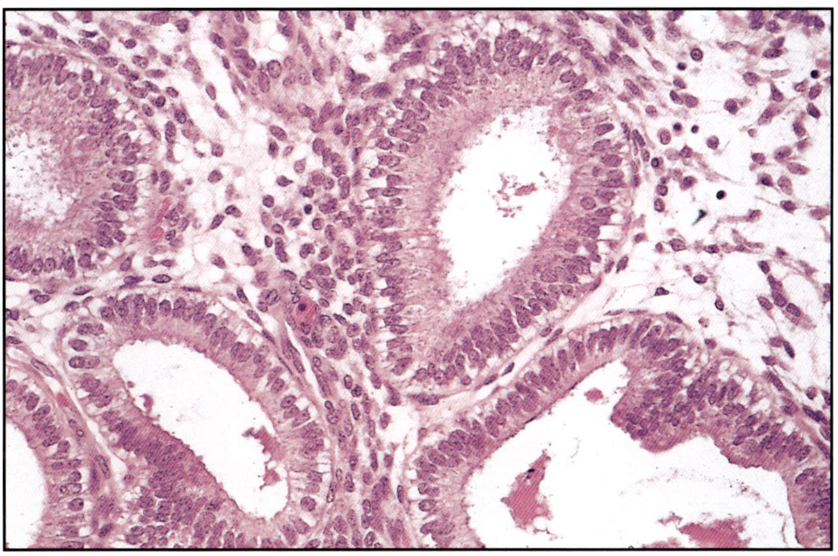

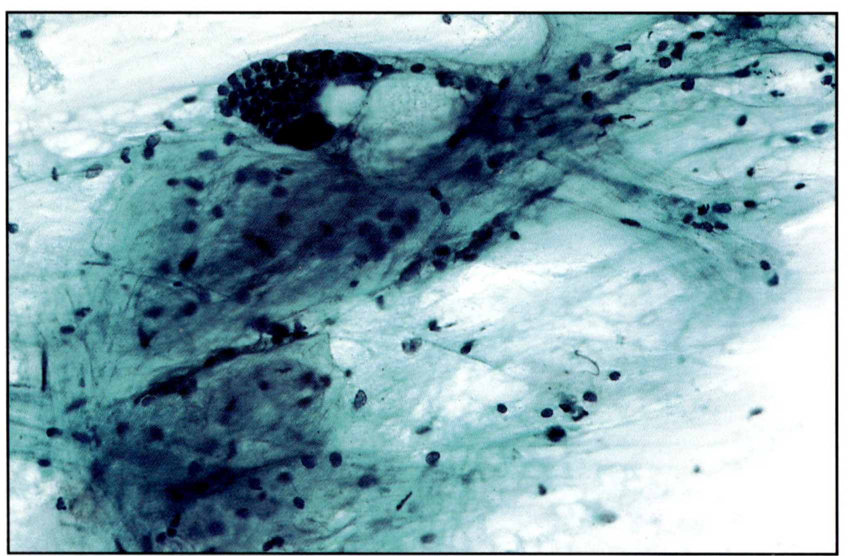

Image 2.56
Endometrium of the midsecretory phase. By the fifth postovulatory day, most of the secretion has been discharged into the glandular lumen, and thus copious thick, mucoid material is noted in direct smear preparations (cannot be appreciated in Cytospin preparations). This finding in an endometrial brushing indicates that the date is at least day 19 of the menstrual cycle (Papanicolaou, 100X).

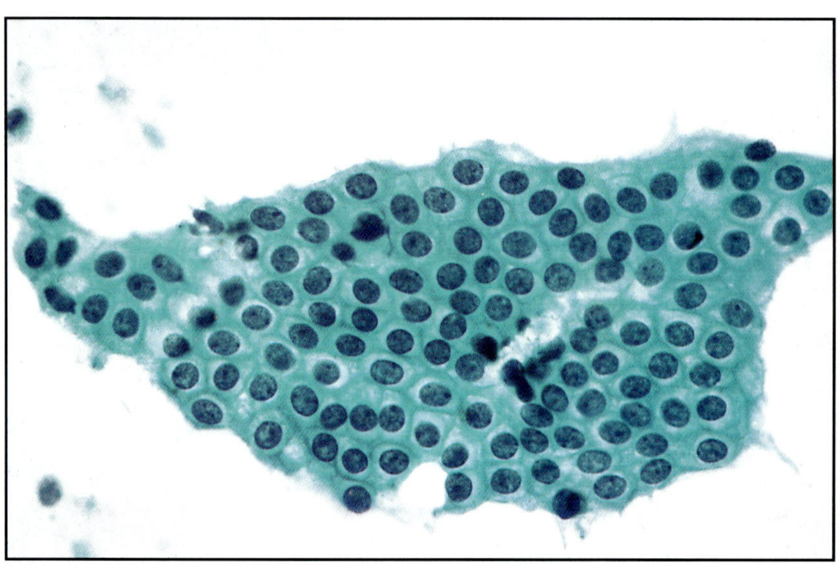

Image 2.57
Endometrium of the midsecretory phase. The secretory glandular cells have an abundance of well-defined clear cytoplasm and large, round or slightly ovoid, vesicular nuclei. They occur in sheet arrangements with a honeycomb pattern. Endometrial brushing (Papanicolaou, 400X).

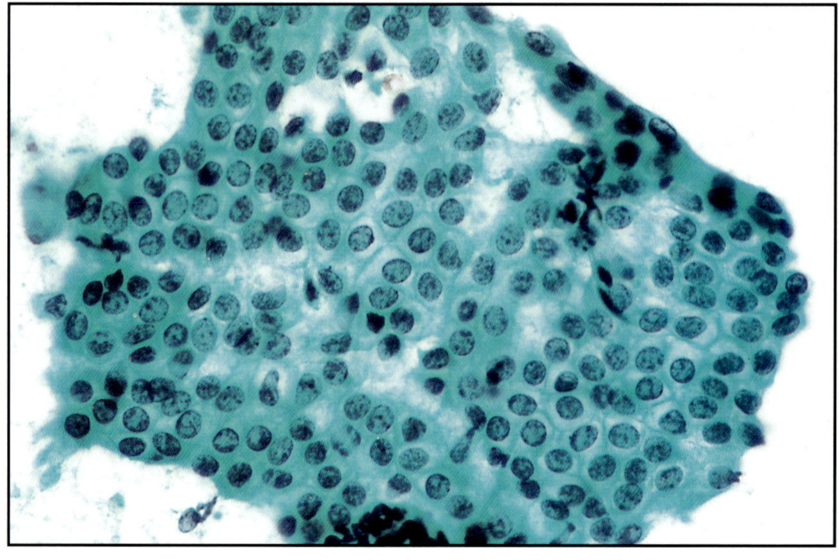

Image 2.58
Endometrium of the midsecretory phase. The nuclei of the secretory glandular cells during this phase, unlike those seen during the early secretory phase (see Images 2.52 and 2.53), become enlarged, rounded, and have a fine chromatin pattern. Occasional small or prominent nucleoli are noted. Endometrial brushing (Papanicolaou, 400X).

Image 2.59
Endometrium of the midsecretory phase. The stromal cells have scant, ill-defined cytoplasm and enlarged, plump, vesicular nuclei with fine chromatin. They occur in loose, non-cohesive groupings. Endometrial brushing (Papanicolaou, 400X).

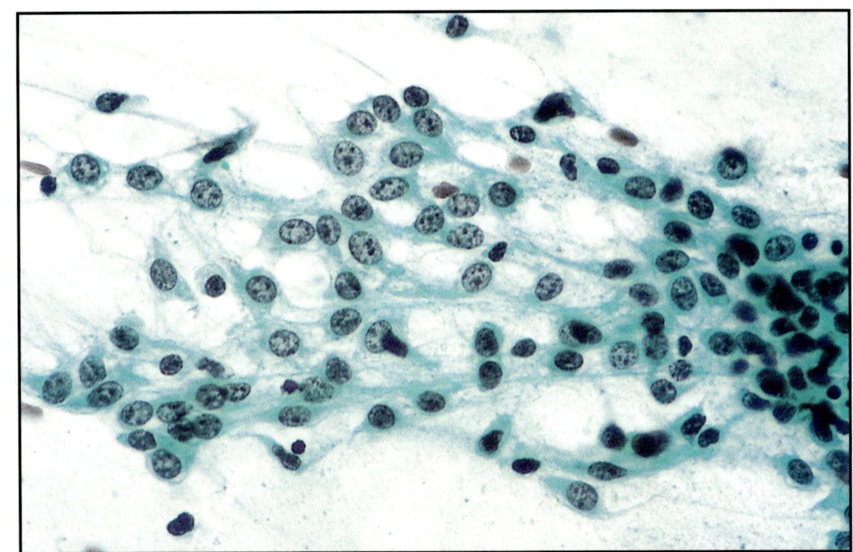

Image 2.60
Endometrium of the midsecretory phase. The caliber of the glands has increased, and the sawtooth appearance of their contours is noted. The glandular cells appear nonvacuolated (clear in brushing preparations), and the glands contain abundant luminal secretion. Histologic section (H&E, 200X).

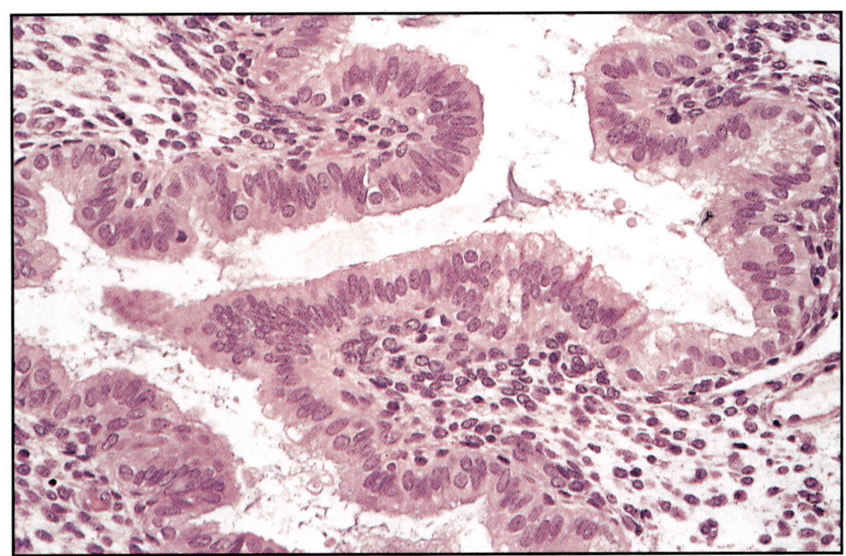

Image 2.61
Endometrium of the late secretory phase. The secretory glandular cells have round or ovoid nuclei with coarse chromatin and a moderate amount of well-defined, somewhat dense cytoplasm. They occur in sheet arrangements with a honeycomb pattern. They probably represent "exhausted" secretory glandular cells (compare these cells with those shown in Image 2.57). Endometrial brushing (Papanicolaou, 400X).

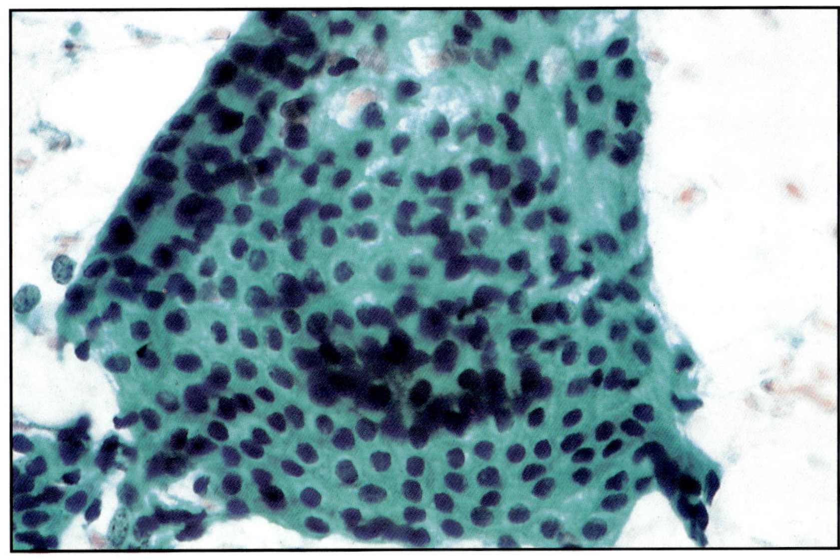

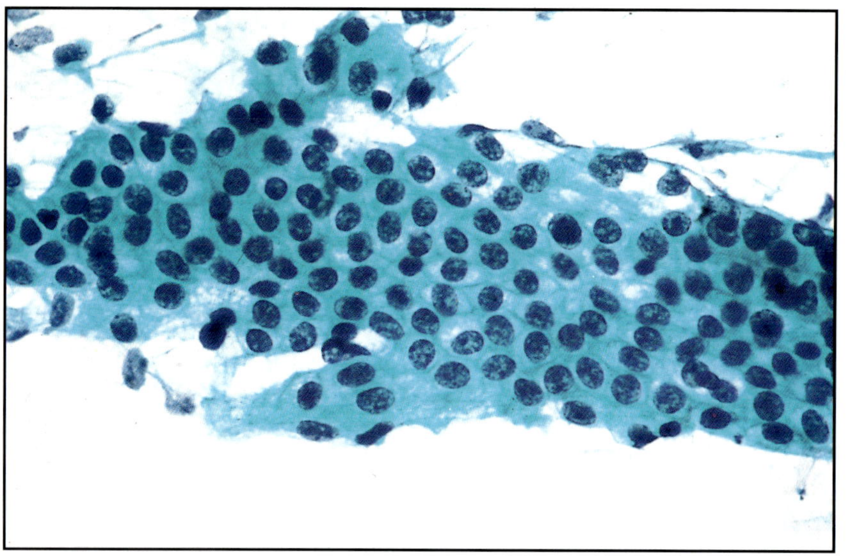

Image 2.62
Endometrium of the late secretory phase. Some of the glandular cells have dense cytoplasm and smaller nuclei with coarse chromatin, and admix with secretory glandular cells that have clear or partially clear cytoplasm and larger nuclei with slightly coarse chromatin. This probably represents different levels of "exhaustion" among glandular cells during this phase. Endometrial brushing (Papanicolaou, 400X).

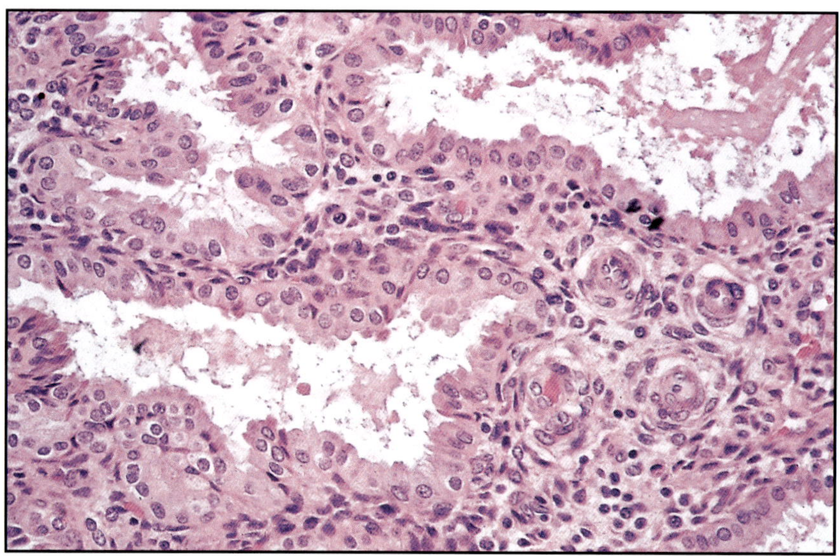

Image 2.63
Endometrium of the late secretory phase. The secretory glands are prominently coiled, have sawtooth contours, and contain abundant luminal secretion. The increased prominence of the spiral arteries is evident. Predecidual changes in perivascular stromal cells are also noted. Histologic section (H&E, 200X).

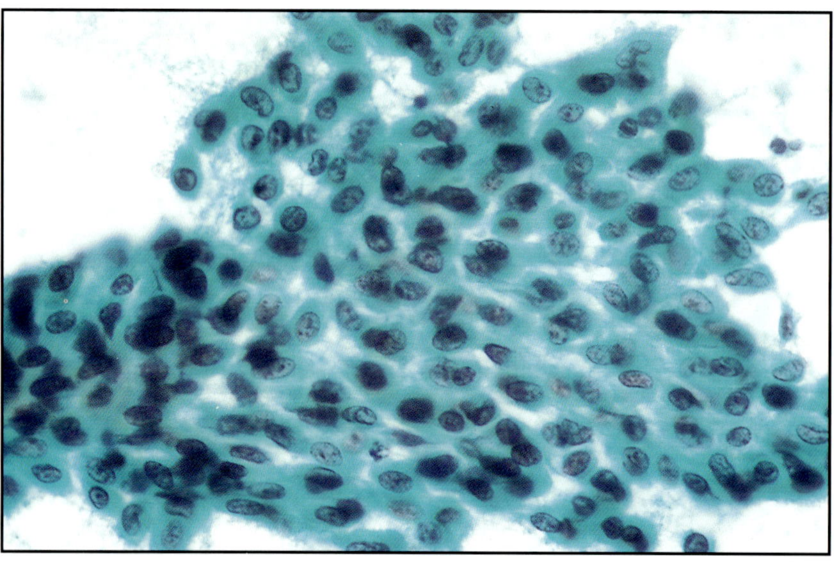

Image 2.64
Endometrium of the late secretory phase. The stromal cells in the upper portion of the endometrium undergo predecidual changes. They acquire more dense or granular cytoplasm and round or ovoid, vesicular nuclei with occasional prominent nucleoli. They occur in a sheet arrangement. Note that the nuclei are variable in size. Endometrial brushing (Papanicolaou, 400X).

Image 2.65
Endometrium of the late secretory phase. Some of the predecidual cells (the predecidualized stromal cells) have an abundance of granular cytoplasm and large ovoid, vesicular nuclei with occasional prominent nucleoli. They admix with small stromal cells (non-predecidualized) that have relatively scant cytoplasm and smaller dense nuclei. Endometrial brushing (Papanicolaou, 400X).

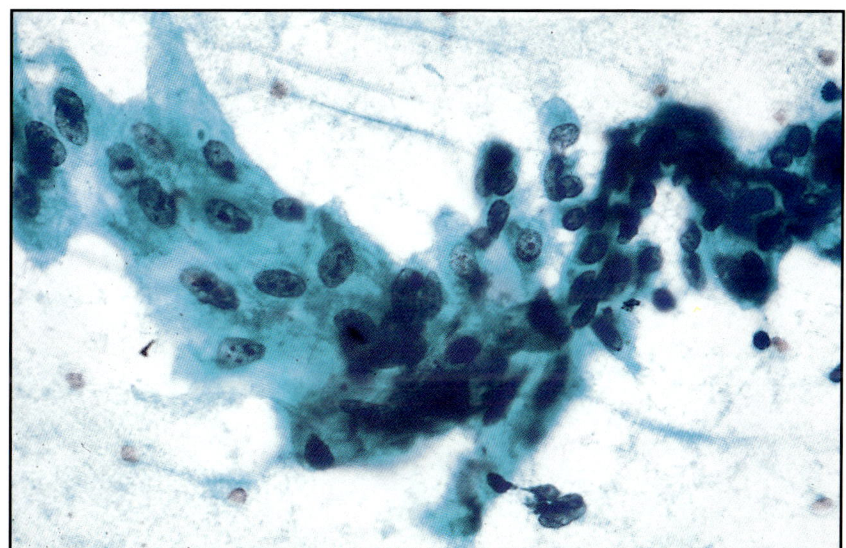

Image 2.66
Endometrium of the late secretory phase. The predecidual cells have an abundance of dense cytoplasm and large vesicular nuclei. They occur in cohesive groupings, mimicking smooth muscle cells from the myometrium. Endometrial brushing (Papanicolaou, 400X).

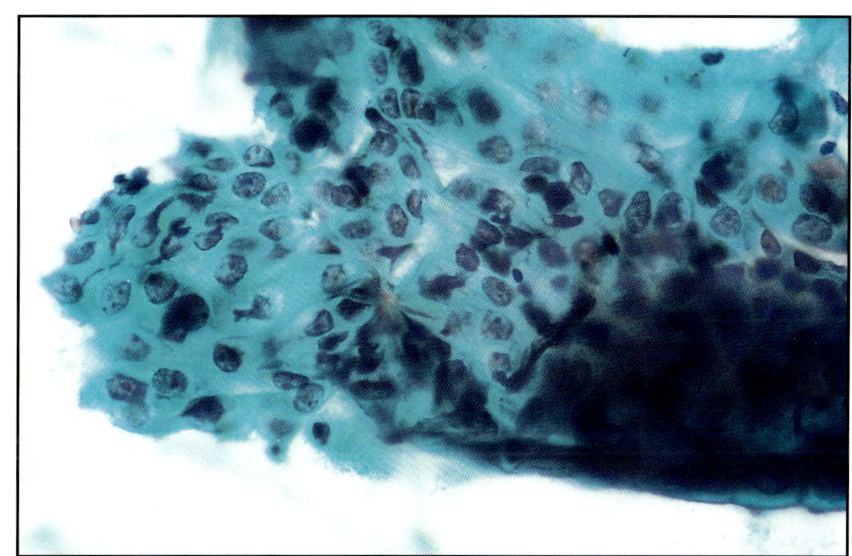

Image 2.67
Endometrium of the late secretory phase. Clusters of predecidual cells with large, round or ovoid nuclei and a moderate amount to an abundance of well-defined, dense cytoplasm are in close proximity to a sheet of "exhausted" secretory glandular cells with smaller round nuclei and a small to moderate amount of somewhat dense or partially clear cytoplasm. Endometrial brushing (Papanicolaou, 400X).

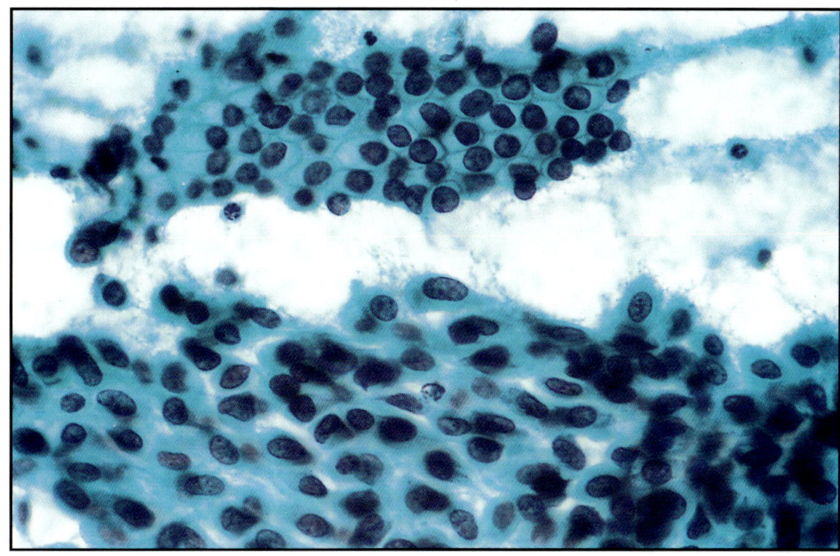

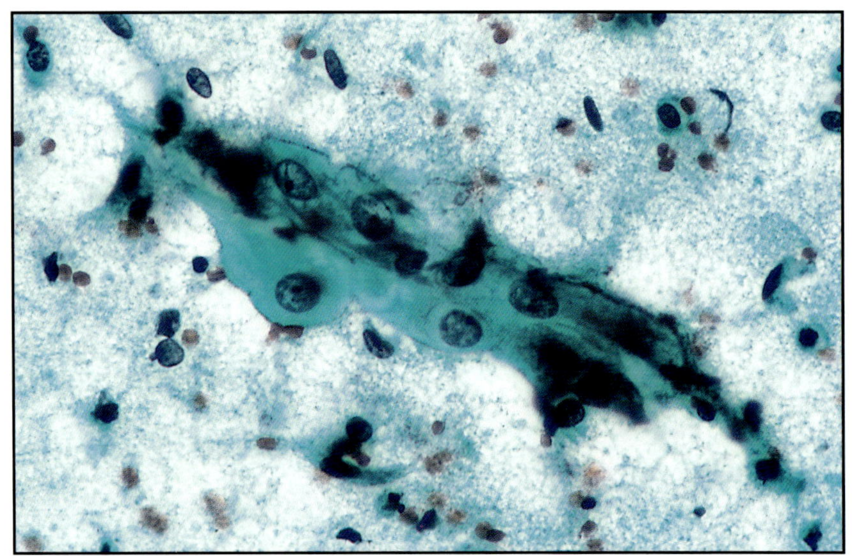

Image 2.68

Endometrium of the late secretory phase. Towards the end of the secretory phase, some of the perivascular predecidual cells reach very large size, resembling decidual cells seen during pregnancy. They have large vesicular nuclei with frequent prominent nucleoli and an abundance of somewhat dense cytoplasm. Endometrial brushing (Papanicolaou, 400X).

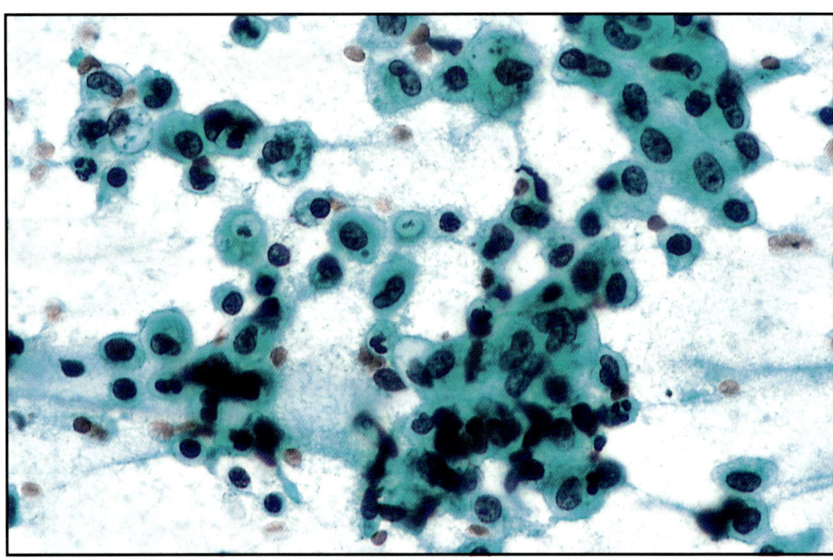

Image 2.69

Endometrium of the late secretory phase. At the end of the secretory phase as the stroma begins to disintegrate, many predecidual cells in the upper portion of the endometrium separate from each other. These solitary predecidual cells are present in the endometrial cavity in large numbers. They have round, ovoid, or bean-shaped nuclei and various amounts of foamy or finely granular cytoplasm. Note that a few endometrial granulocytes are present in the background. Endometrial brushing (Papanicolaou, 400X).

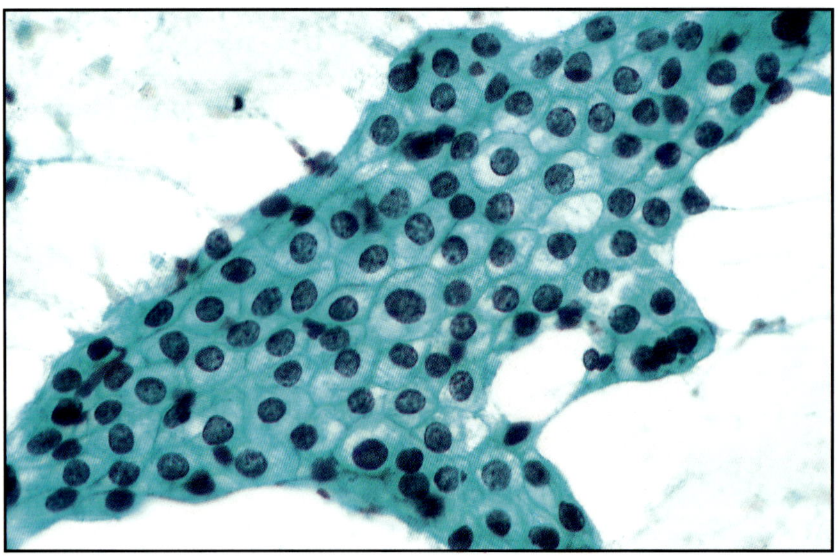

Image 2.70

Endometrium during the early pregnancy. The glandular cells become "exaggerated" secretory cells and are enlarged. They have large, round or ovoid, vesicular nuclei and an abundance of well-defined, clear cytoplasm. They occur in a sheet arrangement with a honeycomb pattern. Endometrial brushing (Papanicolaou, 400X).

Image 2.71
Endometrium during early pregnancy. The very large decidual cells (decidualized stromal cells) have large, round or ovoid, vesicular nuclei with frequent conspicuous nucleoli and an abundance of clear or finely granular cytoplasm. They occur in sheet arrangements. Endometrial brushing (Papanicolaou, 400X).

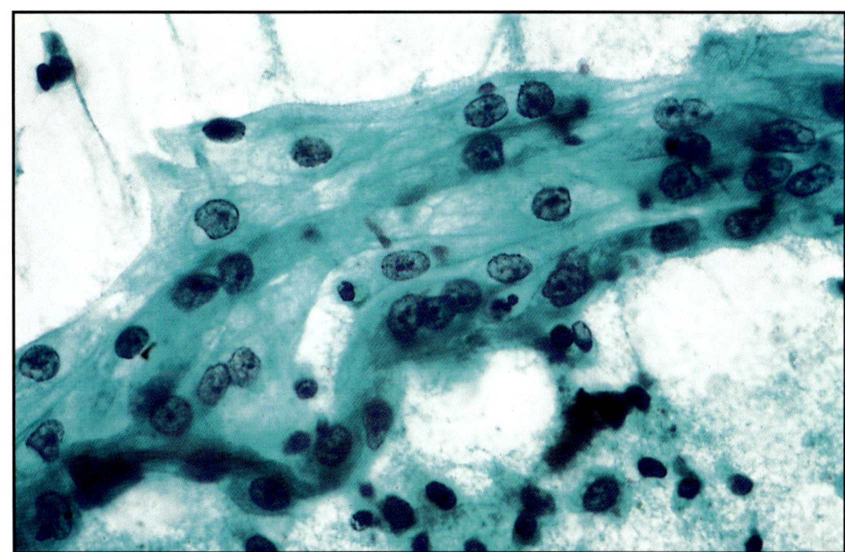

Image 2.72
Endometrium during early pregnancy. The large decidual cells have enlarged, ovoid, vesicular nuclei and an abundance of foamy cytoplasm. They occur in a cohesive grouping. Endometrial brushing (Papanicolaou, 400X).

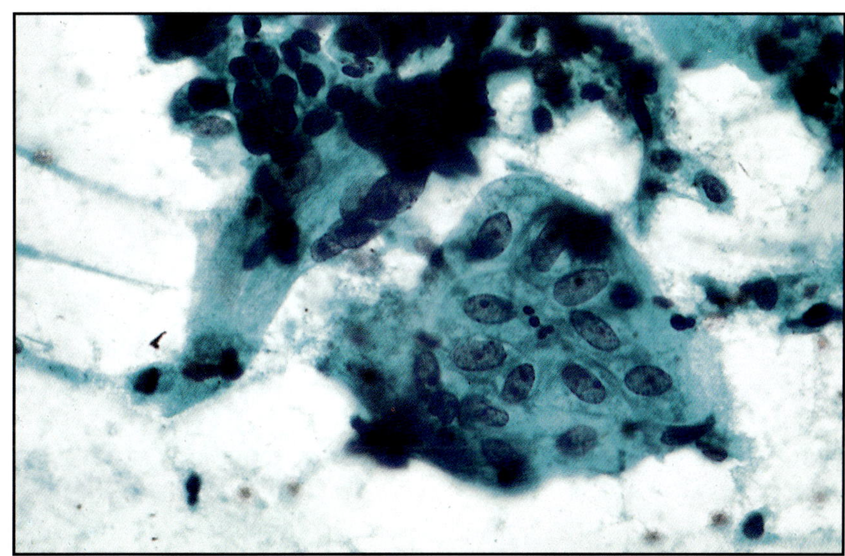

Image 2.73
Endometrium during early pregnancy. The enlarged glands are lined by large secretory cells with abundant vacuolated cytoplasm and surrounded by sheets of very large decidual cells. Histologic section (H&E, 200X).

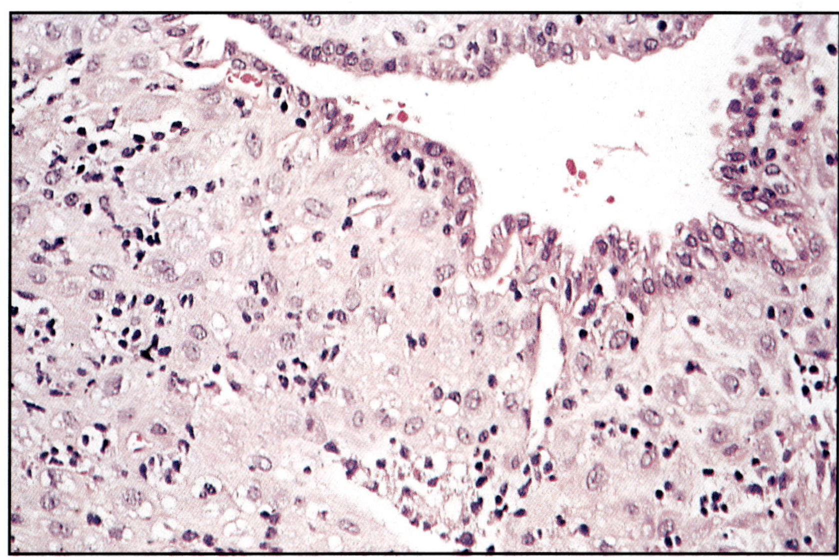

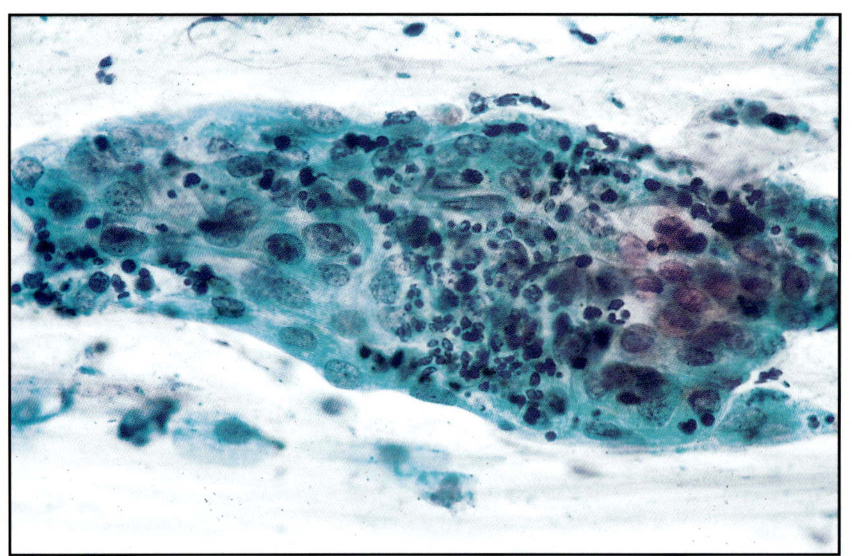

Image 2.74
Endometrium of the menstrual phase. In the center of a menstrual tissue fragment are some glandular cells with rounded nuclei surrounded by large predecidual cells with enlarged, ovoid vesicular nuclei from the upper portion of the endometrium and admixed with leukocytes and nuclear debris. Endometrial brushing (Papanicolaou, 400X).

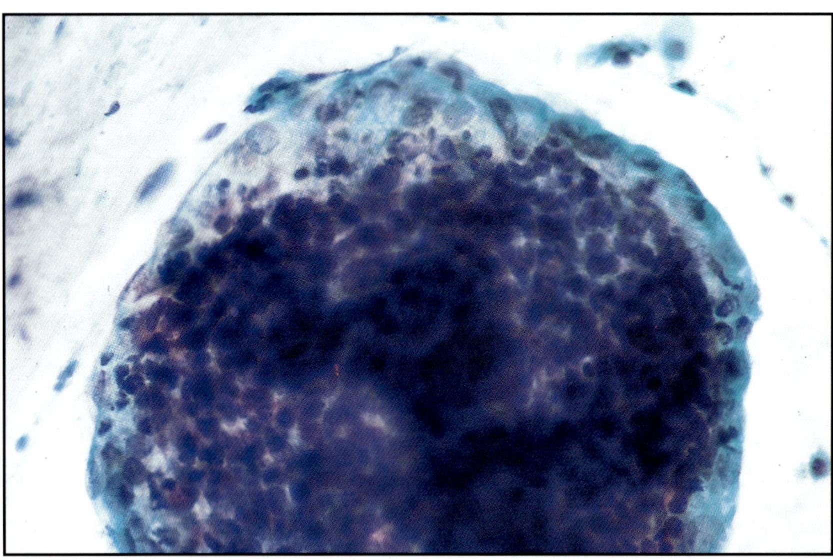

Image 2.75
Endometrium of the menstrual phase. In the center of menstrual tissue fragments are degenerating glandular cells surrounded by large predecidual cells from the upper portion of the endometrium and admixed with leukocytes and nuclear debris. This kind of tissue fragment is often ball-like (or menstrual cell balls), and is only seen during the menstrual phase. Thus, this finding indicates a normal menstrual endometrium. Endometrial brushing (Papanicolaou, 400X).

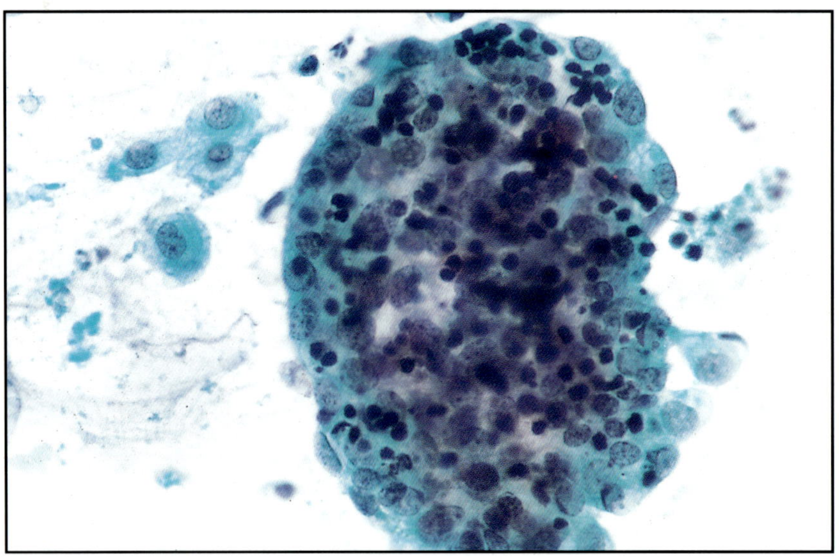

Image 2.76
Endometrium of the menstrual phase. A menstrual cell ball consists of large predecidual cells with enlarged vesicular nuclei and a moderate amount of foamy cytoplasm admixed with leukocytes and nuclear debris. Note that a few solitary predecidual cells are present in the left upper corner. Endometrial brushing (Papanicolaou, 400X).

Image 2.77
Endometrium of the menstrual phase. A menstrual cell ball consists of degenerating glandular and predecidual cells partially surrounded by small stromal cells (non-predecidualized) from the lower portion of the endometrium. Note that the small stromal cells have scant, ill-defined cytoplasm and are closely packed. Endometrial brushing (Papanicolaou, 400X).

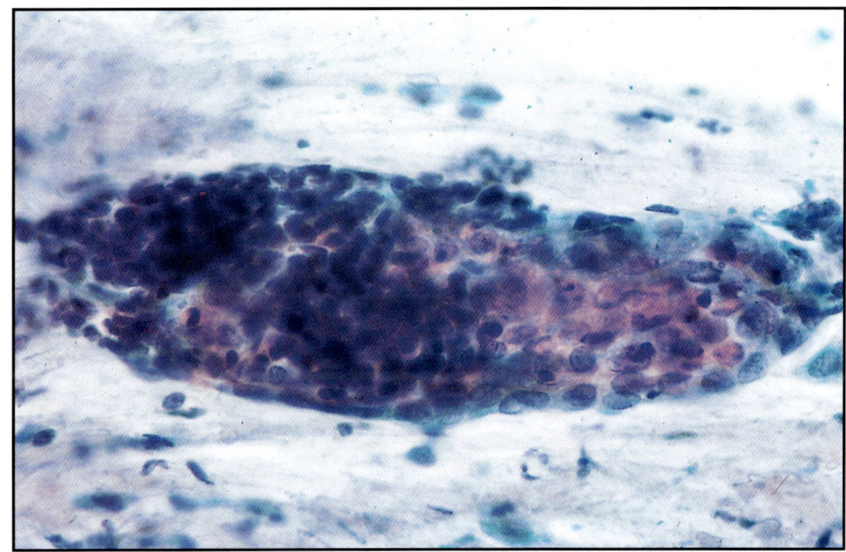

Image 2.78
An exodus of solitary predecidual cells during the menstrual phase. An exodus of numerous solitary predecidual cells that have round, ovoid, or bean-shaped nuclei and various amounts of well-defined, finely granular or foamy cytoplasm is seen in a cervicovaginal smear procured during the menstrual phase (compare these cells with those shown in Image 2.69) (Papanicolaou, 400X).

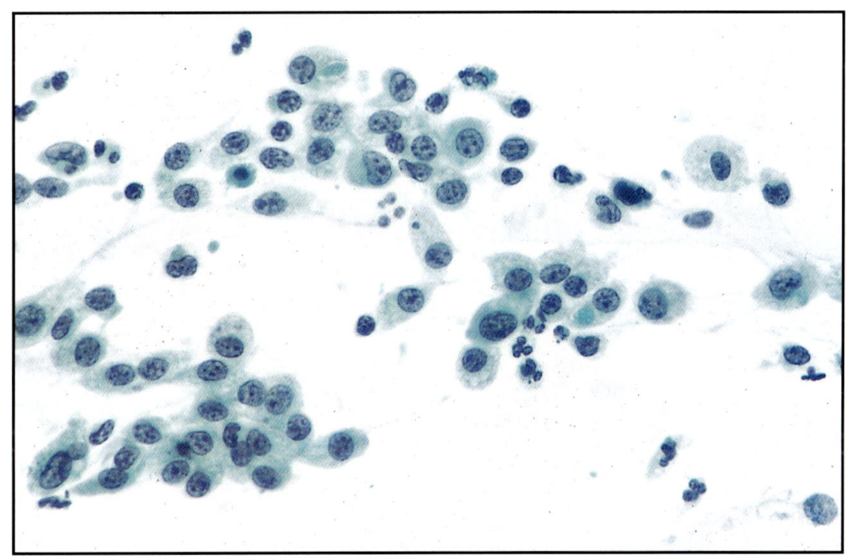

Image 2.79
Atrophic endometrium in a postmenopausal woman. The glandular cells have relatively small, round or ovoid, vesicular nuclei and scant cytoplasm. They occur in sheet arrangements. Nuclear crowding and overlapping are not present. Endometrial brushing (Papanicolaou, 400X).

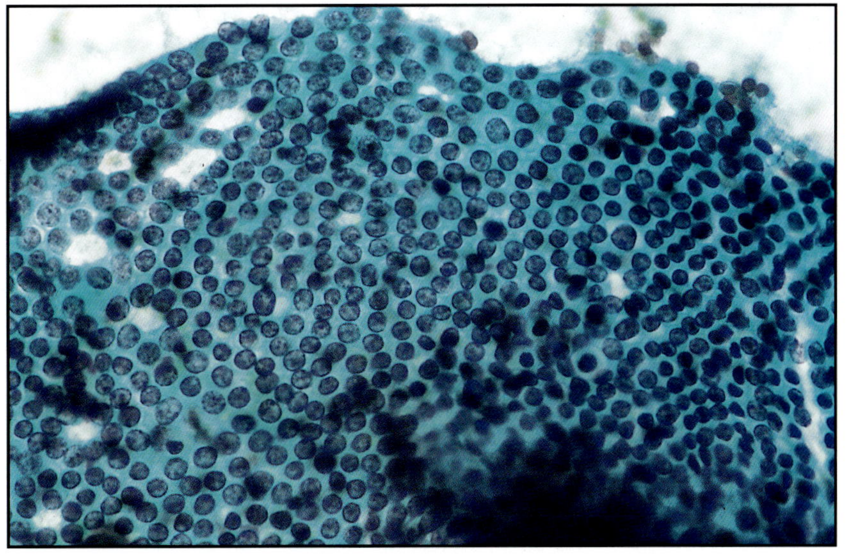

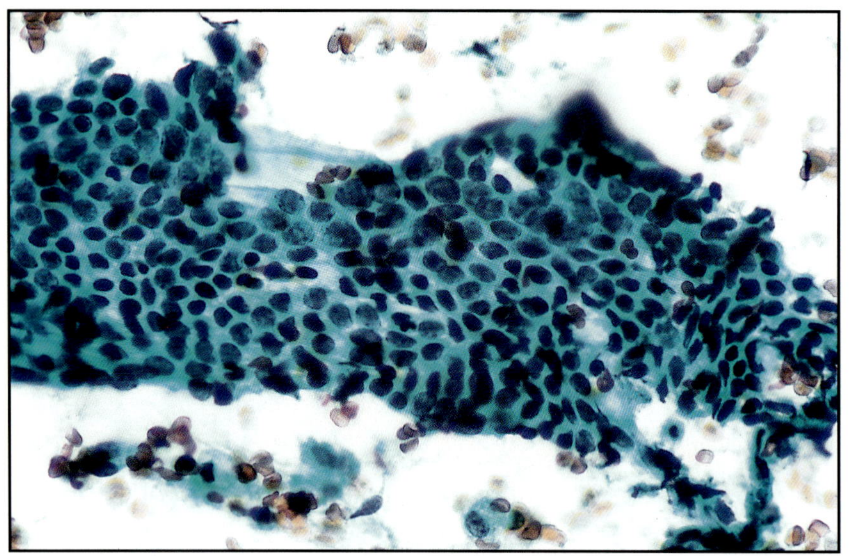

Image 2.80
Atrophic endometrium in a postmeno-pausal woman. The glandular cells have round or ovoid, vesicular nuclei and scant cytoplasm, and admix with glandular cells that have pyknotic nuclei and ill-defined cytoplasm. Endometrial brushing (Papanicolaou, 400X).

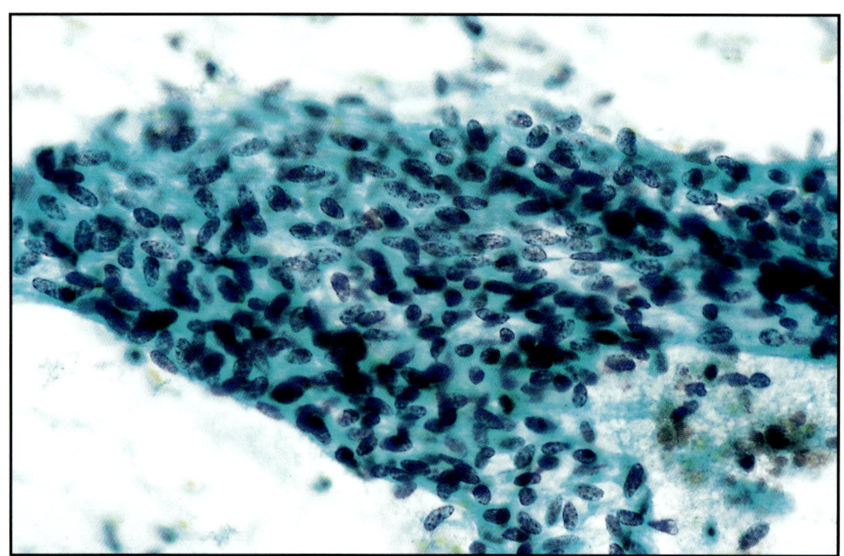

Image 2.81
Atrophic endometrium in a postmeno-pausal woman. The stromal cells have scant, ill-defined cytoplasm and plump, fusiform or pyknotic nuclei. They occur in loose groupings. They are spindled and closely packed. Endo-metrial brushing (Papanicolaou, 400X).

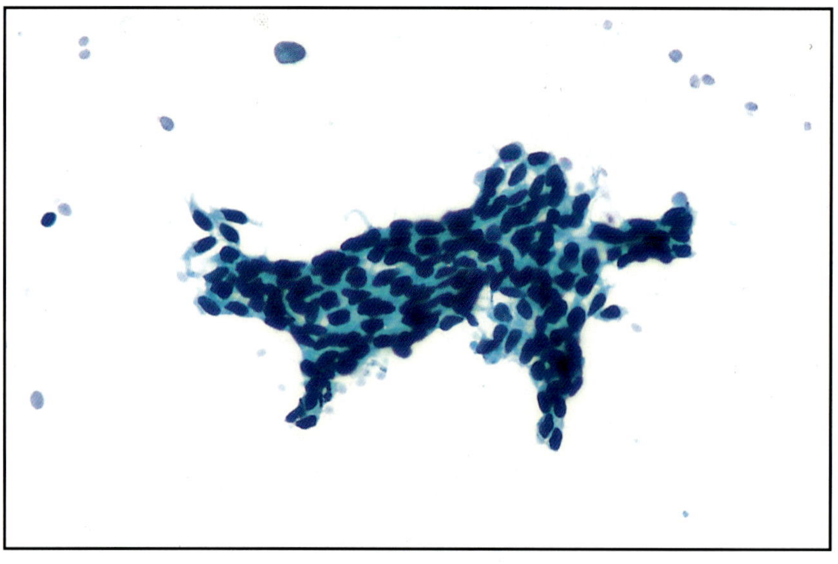

Image 2.82
Atrophic endometrium in a postmeno-pausal woman. The stromal cells have fusiform, pyknotic nuclei and scant, ill-defined cytoplasm. They occur in loose groupings. Endometrial brushing (Papanicolaou, 400X).

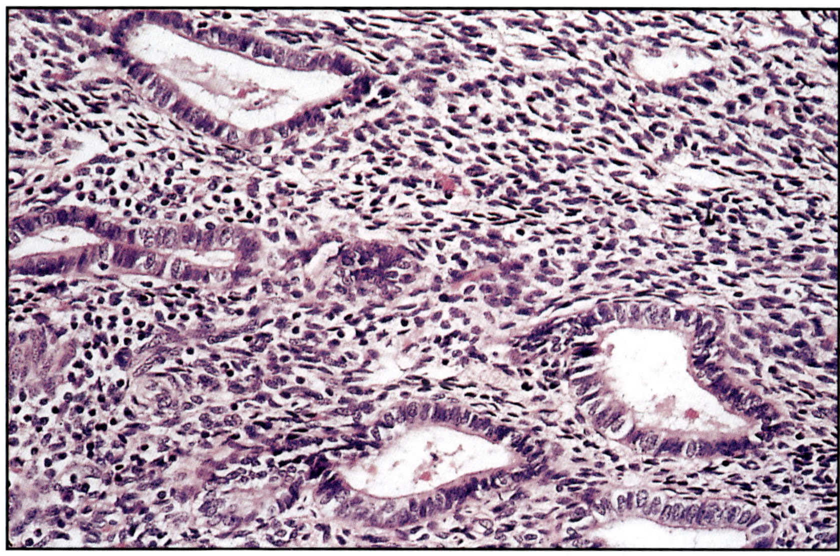

Image 2.83
Atrophic endometrium in a postmenopausal woman. The small glands comprise a single layer of cuboidal or low columnar epithelial cells with scant cytoplasm and occasional pyknotic nuclei. The stromal cells are spindled and have plump, fusiform or pyknotic nuclei. Histologic section (H&E, 200X).

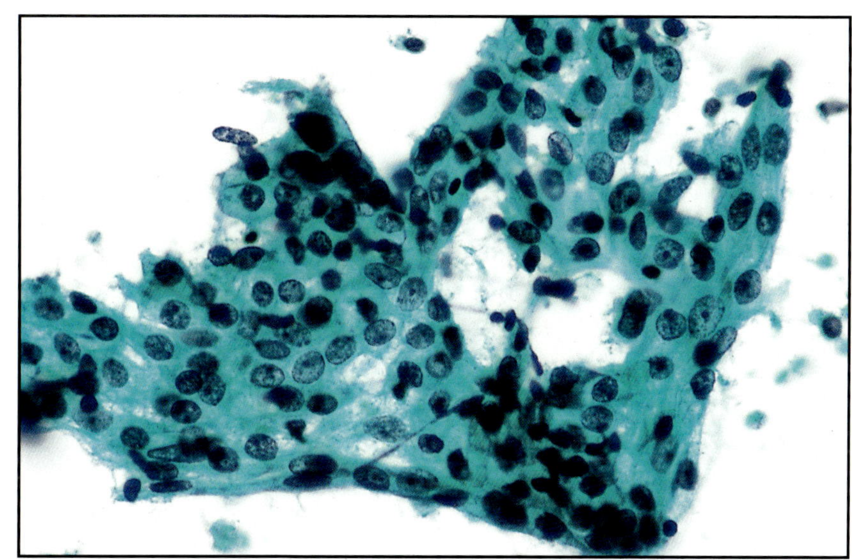

Image 2.84
Atrophic endometrium in a postmenopausal woman taking progestational agents. There are few inactive glandular cells, and numerous stromal cells have a moderate amount of somewhat dense cytoplasm and large vesicular nuclei, resembling predecidual cells seen during the late secretory phase. Endometrial brushing (Papanicolaou, 400X).

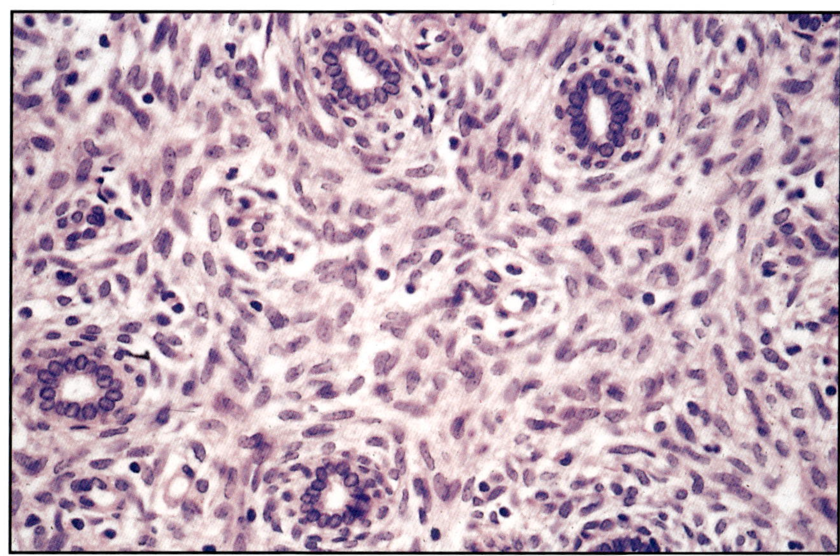

Image 2.85
Atrophic endometrium in a postmenopausal woman taking progestational agents. The glands are small and inactive, and are surrounded by large cells, reminiscent of predecidual cells seen during the late secretory phase. Histologic section (H&E, 200X).

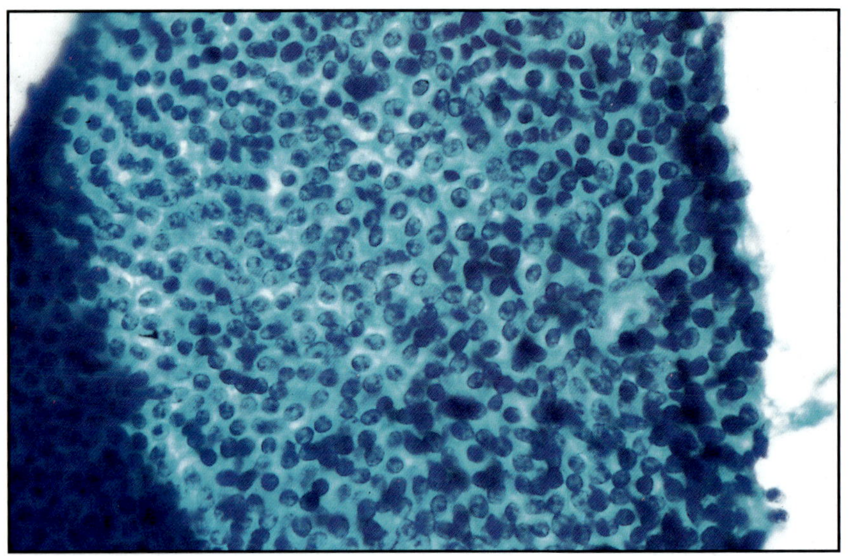

Image 2.86
Weakly proliferative endometrium in a postmenopausal woman. The glandular cells have scant cytoplasm and small ovoid nuclei with fine chromatin. They occur in sheet arrangements. Nuclear crowding is not significant. Endometrial brushing (Papanicolaou, 400X).

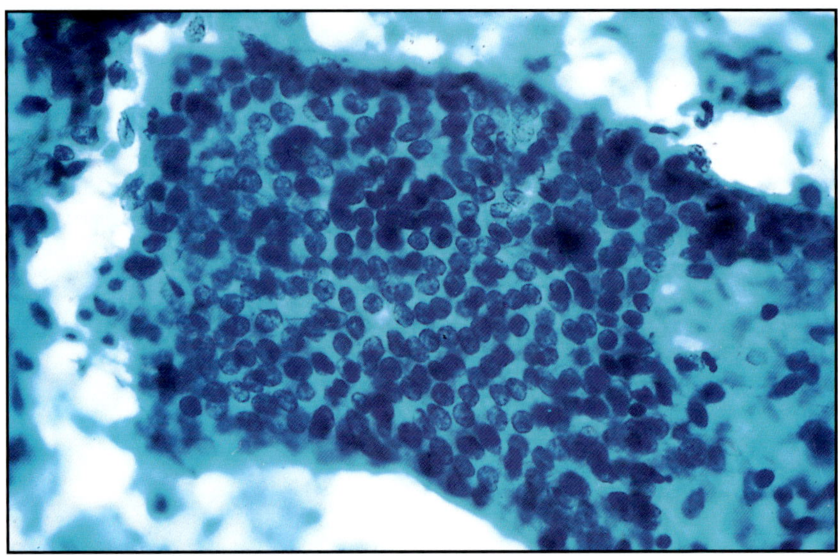

Image 2.87
Weakly proliferative endometrium in a postmenopausal woman. A flat sheet of glandular cells contains uniform and regular, round or ovoid nuclei. The cytologic features are similar to those seen during the early proliferative phase except that the nuclei appear less crowded and mitotic figures are scarce. Endometrial brushing (Papanicolaou, 400X).

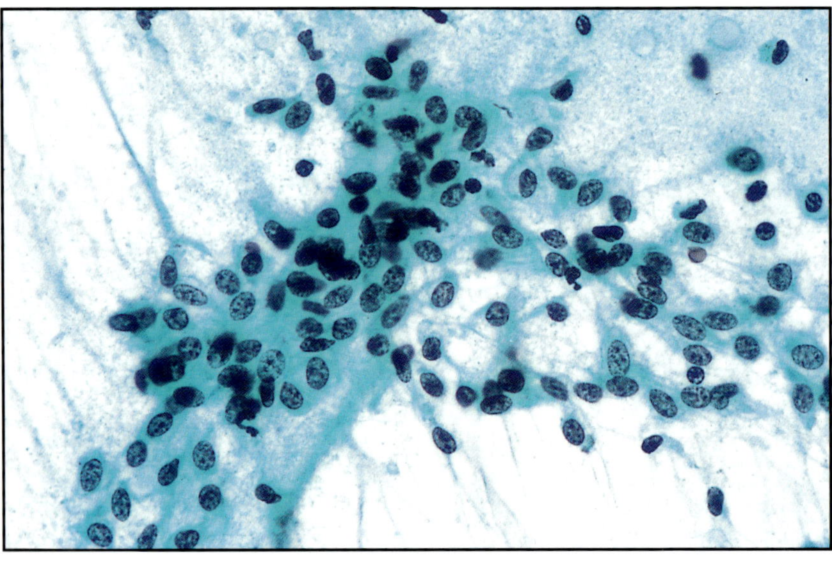

Image 2.88
Weakly proliferative endometrium in a postmenopausal woman. The stromal cells are spindled and loosely packed. They have scant, ill-defined cytoplasm and plump or fusiform nuclei. Endometrial brushing (Papanicolaou, 400X).

Image 2.89
Weakly proliferative endometrium in a postmenopausal woman. The glands are dilated and lined by nonstratified, thin, columnar or cuboidal cells with dense nuclei. Mitotic figures are scarce. The stromal cells are spindled. Histologic section (H&E, 100X).

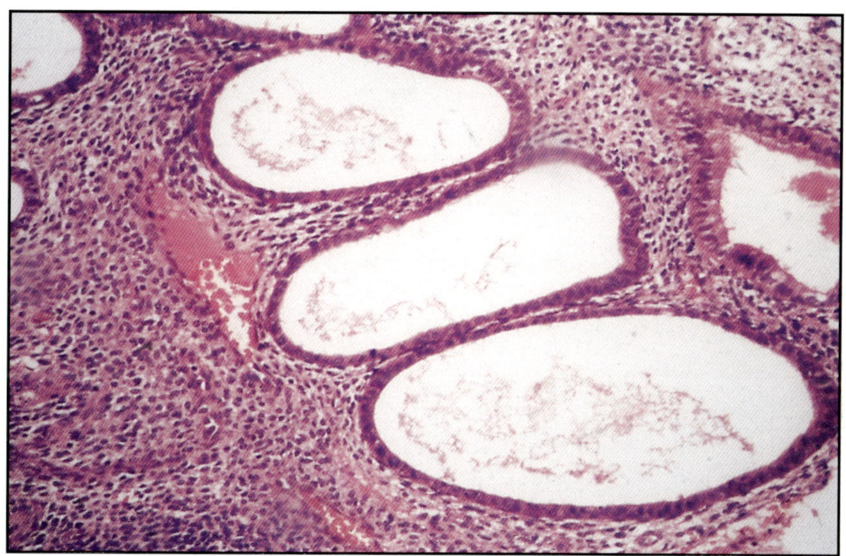

Image 2.90
Disordered proliferative endometrium in a perimenopausal woman. The glandular cells have scant cytoplasm and round or ovoid nuclei with inconspicuous nuclei, and occur in sheet arrangements with nuclear crowding and overlapping. Endometrial brushing (Papanicolaou, 400X).

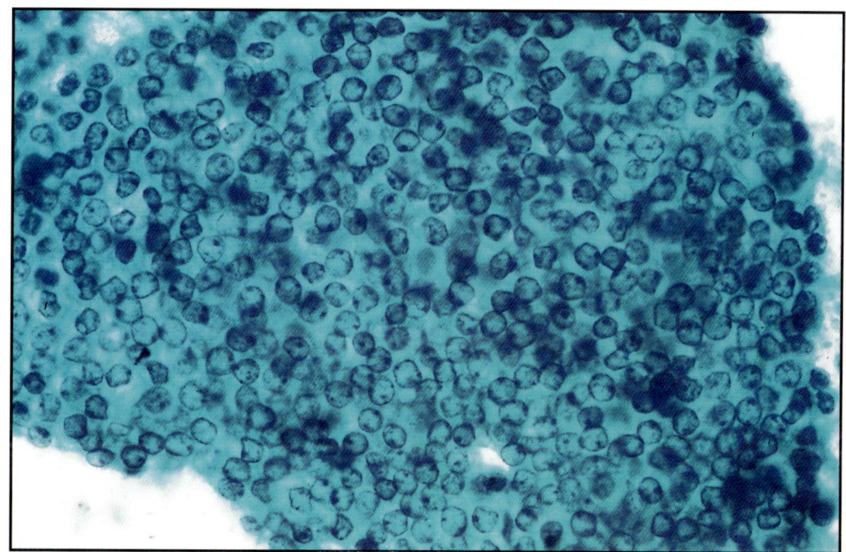

Image 2.91
Disordered proliferative endometrium in a perimenopausal woman. Sheets of crowding glandular cells that have uniform and regular, round or ovoid nuclei with dense chromatin and small nucleoli, and scant cytoplasm resemble flat sheets of glandular cells seen during the proliferative phase in premenopausal women. Endometrial brushing (Papanicolaou, 400X).

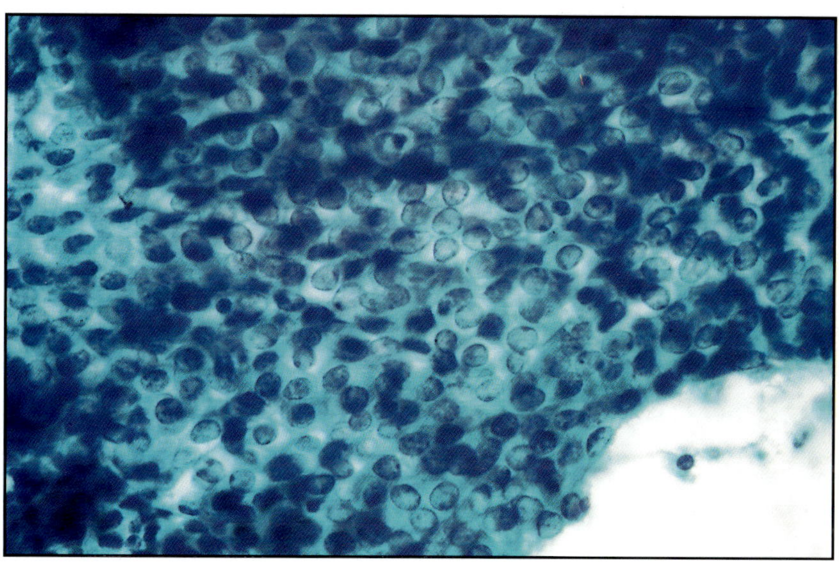

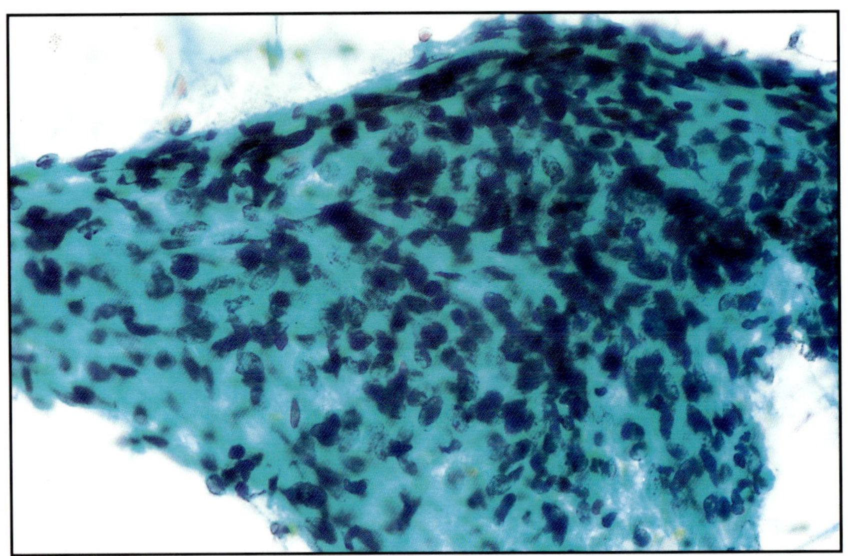

Image 2.92
Disordered proliferative endometrium in a perimenopausal woman. The stromal cells have an abundance of ill-defined cytoplasm and ovoid or fusiform nuclei with slightly dense chromatin, and occur in cohesive groupings. Endometrial brushing (Papanicolaou, 400X).

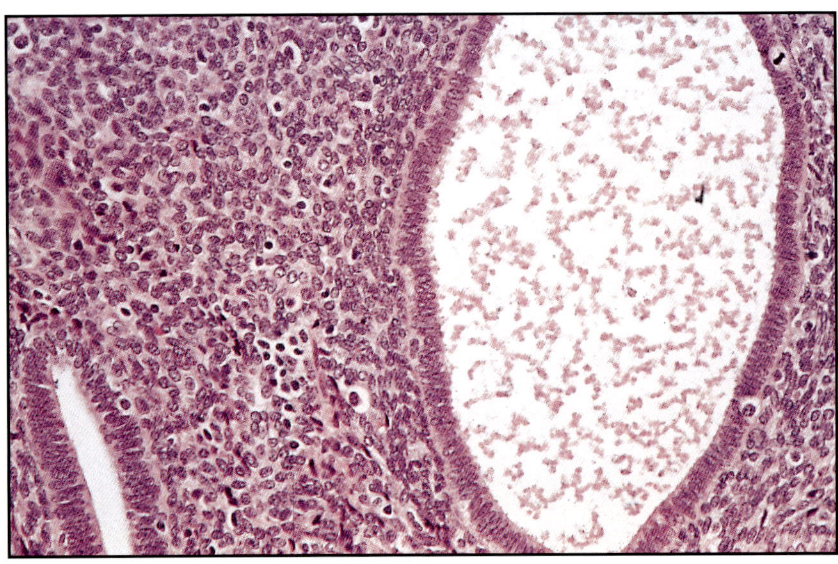

Image 2.93
Disordered proliferative endometrium in perimenopausal woman. The glands are cystically dilated and lined by columnar cells. Pseudostratification of the glandular cells and mitotic figures are present. The stromal cells are spindled and have plump nuclei. Histologic section (H&E, 200X).

References

1. Azzopardi JG, Zayid I: Synthetic progestogen-estrogen therapy and uterine changes. *J Clin Pathol* 20:731–738, 1967.

2. Dallenbach FD, Rudolph HG: Foam cells and estrogen activity of the human endometrium. *Arch Gynecol* 217:335–347, 1974.

3. Dallenbach-Hellweg G: *Histopathology of the Endometrium.* New York, NY, Springer-Verlag NY Inc, 1981.

4. Denholm RB, More IA: Atypical cilia of the human endometrial epithelium. *J Anat* 131:309–315, 1980.

5. Elwood MJ, Cole P, Rothman KJ, et al: Epidemiology of endometrial cancer. *J Natl Cancer Inst* 59:1055–1060, 1977.

6. Fechner RE, Bossarl MI, Spjut R: Ultrastructure of endometrial stromal foam cells. *Am J Clin Pathol* 72:628–633, 1979.

7. Fritz MA, Speroff L: The endocrinology of the menstrual cycle: The interaction of folliculogenesis and neuroendocrine mechanisms. *Fertil Steril* 38:509–529, 1982.

8. Hendricken MR, Kempson RL: Uterus and fallopian tube. In: *Histology for Pathologists,* Sternberg SS (editor). New York, NY, Raven Press, 1992, pp 797–826.

9. Hodgen GD: Neuroendocrinology of the normal menstrual cycle. *J Reprod Med* 34:68–75, 1982.

10. Kearns M, Lala PK: Life history of decidual cells: A review. *Am J Reprod Immunol* 3:78–82, 1983.

11. Koss LG: *Diagnostic Cytology and Its Histologic Bases.* 4th ed. Philadelphia, PA, JB Lippincott Co, 1992, pp 535–587.

12. Koss, LG, Schreiber K, Moussouris H, et al: Endometrial carcinoma and its precursors: Detection and screening. *Clin Obstet Gynecol* 25:49–61, 1982.

13. McBride JM: The normal postmenopausal endometrium. *J Obstet Gynecol Br Emp* 61:691–697, 1954.

14. Nogales-Ortiz F, Puerta J, Nogales FF Jr: The normal menstrual cycle: Chronology and mechanism of endometrial desquamation. *Obstet Gynecol* 51:259–264, 1978.

15. Ober WB: Effects of oral and intrauterine administration of contraceptives on the uterus. *Hum Pathol* 8:513–527, 1977.

16. Palermo V: Interpretation of endometrium obtained by the Endo-Pap sampler and a clinical study of its use. *Diagn Cytopathol* 1:5–12, 1985.

17. Parks RD, Scheerer PP, Greene RR: The endometria of normal postmenopausal women. *Surg Gynecol Obstet* 106:413–420, 1958.

18. Reagan JW, Ng ABP: *The Cells of Uterine Adenocarcinoma.* New York, NY, S Karger, 1973, pp 7–24.

19. Schueller EF: Ciliated epithelia of the human uterine mucosa. *Obstet Gynecol* 31:215–223, 1968.

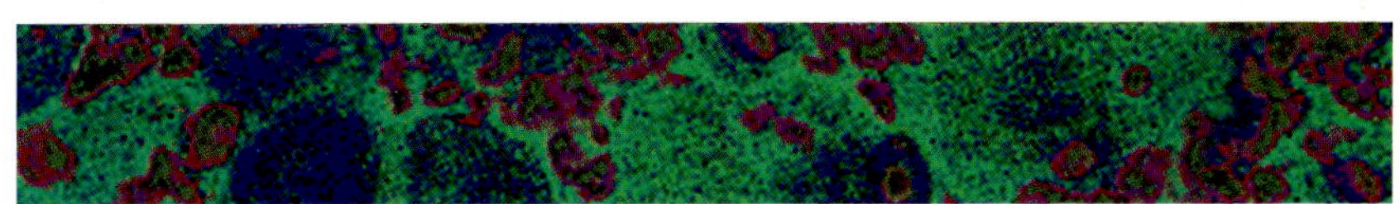

CHAPTER THREE

Benign Disorders of the Endometrium

The uterus is stimulated daily by hormones and denuded monthly of its endometrial mucosa. As a result of this cyclic change, the endometrium is remarkably resistant to infection. Acute reactions are virtually limited to bacterial infections that arise following delivery or miscarriage. Retained products of conception are the usual predisposing influence. Removal of the retained gestational fragments by curettage is promptly followed by remission of the infection. In the majority of cases, the causative organism is a streptococcus, a staphylococcus, a colibacillus, an enterococcus (principally in puerperal infection), a gonococcus, or a tubercle bacillus. Regardless of the cause of the histologic type of endometritis, the endometrial glands respond to the inflammation in a manner that is totally independent of endogenous hormonal stimuli. Thus, mixed phase patterns are usually seen, and the glands often show reactive hyperplasia, which is a pitfall in the interpretation of endometrial cytologic preparations. Neoplastic conditions, such as leiomyoma and polyp, infertility disorders, and other nonneoplastic conditions, such as squamous metaplasia and irradiation changes, which both are sources of diagnostic error in the cytologic interpretation, will also be discussed in this chapter.

Acute Endometritis

Acute endometritis occurs as an ascending infection when the cervical barrier is damaged and is seen usually in association with abortion, instrumentation, or postpartum. Gonococcal endometritis is rarely encountered in our practice because of its very transient nature. The histologic diagnosis of acute endometritis is based on finding aggregates of neutrophils in the stroma, forming microabscesses and filling the glandular lumens. The cyclic function of the endometrium is often preserved. The infected portions of the endometrium may be shed with the menstruation unless the basal layer is also involved. The term pyometra designates the accumulation of pus within the endometrial cavity, and is the consequence of the combined effect of obstruction and infection. The most common cause of obstruction is the result of cervical stricture originating from senile atresia, surgery, cauterization, irradiation, uterine prolapse, or cervical or endometrial carcinoma.[11] The causative organisms are the common pyogens, but frequently the infection is a mixed one. The inflammatory reaction is usually confined to the endometrium and immediately adjacent myometrium. The surface and glandular epithelia are more or less destroyed by the heavy inflammatory infiltrates, and the reticulin fibers of the stroma disintegrate. There are areas of hemorrhage and/or edema in the stroma. *Chlamydia trachomatis* has also been identified as a cause of endometritis with increasing frequency in recent years.

In endometrial brushing preparations, there are abundant neutrophils intermixed with glandular cells and stromal cells (Images 3.1 and 3.2). Lymphocytes and occasional plasma cells are also seen. Necrotic debris may be noticed in some cases. When purulent material is obtained, the specimen is also sent for microbiologic studies to identify the causative organisms. If no malignant cells are identified in the endometrial samples, and malignancy is suspected clinically, repeated brushing after the pus is drained is recommended.

Chronic Endometritis

Chronic inflammation of the endometrium may follow abortion or pregnancy, or be the result of wearing an intrauterine contraceptive device. It may be associated with mucopurulent cervicitis and/or pelvic inflammatory disease.[9,10] Endometritis can only become chronic when the endometrium does not shed with menstruation. The causative agents are the same as in acute endometritis. The most common symptoms are pelvic pain and vaginal bleeding. Chronic endometritis is characterized by an infiltrate of lymphocytes and plasma cells, which are scattered diffusely throughout the stroma or aggregated focally. They also infiltrate and may destroy the surface and glandular epithelia. However, there is no destruction of reticulin fibers of the stroma, and the endometrial architecture is preserved. It must be emphasized that lymphoid follicles, with or without germinal centers, are a normal occurrence in the functionalis of the endometrium and should not be taken as evidence of chronic endometritis. The presence of plasma cells, therefore, constitutes the most important criterion in diagnosing chronic endometritis.[2,10] However, plasma cells may be scant and difficult to identify in some instances. In general, if there is an absence of a normal cyclic pattern, inflammatory cells in the glandular lumens, a focal mononuclear infiltrate, dense stroma, or foci of necrosis or calcification, the possibility of chronic endometritis should be suspected and a search for plasma cells undertaken.

In endometrial brushing preparations, the diagnostic finding, like the criterion used in the histologic diagnosis, is the presence of variable numbers of lymphocytes, plasma cells, and macrophages (Images 3.3–3.6). Whenever there are admixtures of glandular cells or stromal cells and inflammatory cells in the same cell clusters and necrotic and/or calcified debris in the cytologic specimens, chronic endometritis is suspected, and one should look for plasma cells. The glandular cells seen in this condition often show reactive hyperplasia with nuclear atypia.

Granulomatous Endometritis

Endometrial tuberculosis is the most significant cause of granulomatous inflammation of the endometrium. Although it is uncommon in the United States, it is still common in other parts of the world.[7] The development of endometrial tuberculosis is related to that of pulmonary tuberculosis. Endometrial tuberculosis is often asymptomatic, and is discovered in the course of a routine gynecologic examination often performed because of sterility.[3,6] The microscopic diagnosis is based on the identification of acid-fast bacilli in tubercles or culture. The microscopic appearance is characterized by the presence of a granuloma rich in epithelioid cells surrounded by lymphocytes, and containing Langhans giant cells in variable numbers. There may be caseous necrosis of the endometrium and ulceration of the endometrial surface. The tubercles are often found throughout the endometrium. The extent of the involvement of the endometrium by tuberculosis may vary greatly. The glandular epithelium often responds by atypical proliferation, stratification, metaplasia, and/or new gland formation. On histologic sections, atypical glandular epithelial proliferation may be marked. The endometrial function is disturbed, and the peritubercular fibrosis inhibits endometrial shedding. Other rare causes of granulomatous endometritis include fungal and mycoplasmal infections, schistosomiasis (relatively common in other parts of the world where the disease is endemic), enterobiasis, sarcoidosis, and foreign body reactions (eg, after hysterosalpingography).

In endometrial brushing preparations from endometrial tuberculosis, abundant acute and chronic inflammatory cells, epithelioid cells, Langhans-type giant cells, and fibroblasts are present (Images 3.7 and 3.8). Dust-like caseous necrotic debris may be seen. The endometrial samples are usually highly cellular. Acid-fast bacilli are often easier to find in cytologic preparations than on histologic sections. Occasional sheets of large, atypical (reactive) glandular cells with nuclear variation and hyperchromasia suggestive of malignancy may be noticed.[8] However, the overall finding is that of a granulomatous inflammatory process, and is not consistent with an endometrial carcinoma. Cytomorphologic differential diagnosis is necessary from other granulomatous inflammation. Sarcoidosis contains no acid-fast bacilli and shows no caseous necrotic debris. In mycotic or parasitic granulomas, fungal organisms or parasites can often be found. Foreign body granulomas often can be recognized by their birefringent material under polarizing illumination or by the presence of numerous mononuclear and multinucleate lipid-laden macrophages.

Squamous Metaplasia

Squamous metaplasia may be seen in the normal or hyperplastic endometrium. It is sometimes seen in association with uterine polyps.[1] Most cases of squamous metaplasia of the endometrium are seen in premenopausal women, especially in those receiving exogenous estrogens and in those having polycystic ovarian disease. Squamous metaplasia of the endometrium usually appears as nonkeratinizing squamoid cells located either diffusely[4] or in the form of berry-like aggregates (morules).[5] Squamous cells in berry-like aggregates in the superficial layer of the endometrium may also be seen in wearers of intrauterine contraceptive devices. This change should be distinguished from well-differentiated endometrial adenocarcinoma with squamous metaplasia in which the glandular element is malignant.

In endometrial cytologic specimens collected by unprotected sampling devices, such as Endo-Pap and Mi-Mark Endometrial Sampler, metaplastic squamous cells may be contaminants from the cervix. It may not be possible to establish this diagnosis if such devices are used to procure endometrial samples. However, in endometrial brushing preparations procured by the IUMC Endometrial Sampler, the metaplastic squamous cells intermingle with endometrial glandular cells, or sheets of metaplastic squamous cells are in continuity with sheets of glandular cells, indicating squamous metaplasia of the endometrium (Images 3.9 and 3.10).

Irradiation Changes

Irradiation of the normal endometrium, as in the course of radiotherapy of cervical or endometrial cancer, produces atrophy of the endometrial glandular epithelia and bizarre atypical cells with nuclear pleomorphism and pyknosis in the stroma. Cystic degeneration of the stroma is common, and the cystic cavities are often lined by atypical cells with squamoid appearance, probably of mesenchymal origin. The stroma is also infiltrated by leukocytes. If the dose of the radiation is high, necrosis of endometrium may dominate.

In endometrial brushing preparations, irradiation changes are different from those changes seen in cervicovaginal smears, which usually involve squamous epithelial cells. In the endometrial samples, the origin of the affected cells are usually stromal or mesenchymal. The affected cells are enlarged and bizarre-looking with pleomorphic, dense or pyknotic nuclei and an abundance of cytoplasm, cytomorphologically mimicking malignant cells. However, their nuclear/cytoplasmic ratios are not increased. These affected cells occur as solitary cells or in noncohesive groupings. Some of them appear spindled, and have enlarged, pleomorphic, hyperchromatic or pyknotic nuclei, mimicking a sarcoma. Others have large pyknotic nuclei and a moderate amount of well-defined dense cytoplasm, mimicking squamous cell carcinoma. However, their overall cytologic findings do not fit into cytomorphologic appearances of any malignant tumors seen in this area. In addition, they often intermix with recognizable benign cells of stromal origin in the same cell groupings, indicating their benign nature (Images 3.11–3.15).

Endometrial Polyp

The large majority of endometrial polyps are not true neoplasms but probably represent circumscribed foci of hyperplasia. At first, a polyp usually has a broad base. When the surrounding endometrium is repeatedly shed with menstruation, the base of the polyp, which is unresponsive to hormonal stimulation during the menstrual cycle, gradually becomes a slim stalk. Polyps may occur at any age, but are more common in the fifth decade. They may be single or multiple. The glands may be lined by an active pseudostratified epithelium containing mitotic figures and usually show some degree of cystic change. In the postmenopausal patient, the glands may be lined by a flat, inactive glandular epithelium. The stroma of a polyp is composed of spindled, fibroblast-like cells, and contain abundant extracellular fibrous connective tissue. The glands and stroma of the endometrial polyp are unresponsive to hormonal stimulation during the menstrual cycle. Thus, specimens from the polyps may contain endometrium that may be atrophic or weakly proliferative despite a fully proliferative or secretory pattern in the surrounding nonpolypoid endometrium. The diagnosis of endometrial polyp is made on the gross features of the lesion rather than on the microscopic pattern of glands and stroma. It is difficult or even impossible to make a diagnosis of endometrial polyp on a curettage specimen or in an endometrial brushing preparation.

Leiomyoma of the Uterus

Leiomyomas of the uterus are present in 40% of women over 50 years of age

Leiomyomas of the uterus are very common neoplasms. In 40% of women over the age of 50 years, leiomyomas are present in the uterus. They are much more common in blacks. These tumors occur intramurally, directly beneath the endometrium, or subserosally. They may fill the endometrial cavity and emerge from the cervical os as polypoid growths. They may become large enough to block the uterus or cause inflammatory complications.

Histologically, leiomyomas are formed by interlacing bundles of smooth muscle cells separated by well-vascularized connective tissue. It is difficult to make a diagnosis of leiomyoma when only a few small fragments of smooth muscle are present in a curettage specimen. In endometrial brushing preparations, tumor cells have ovoid or blunt-ended elongated nuclei and an abundance of ill-defined cytoplasm, giving a syncytial appearance. The tumor cells from a leiomyoma do not show any cytomorphologic difference from smooth muscle cells of the myometrium, and, therefore, a definitive diagnosis of leiomyoma of the uterus cannot be made by cytologic techniques (Images 3.16 and 3.17). However, the cytologic diagnosis of leiomyoma in other sites can be readily established by fine needle aspiration technique, and the cytologic differentiation between leiomyoma and low-grade leiomyosarcoma is also possible (see Chapter 6).

Infertility Disorders

The conditions that will be discussed in this section are those in which a lack of normal cycling (including noncycling and abnormally cycling disorders) is distinctly pathologic. These disorders are usually associated either with infertility or with dysfunctional uterine bleeding, which refers to abnormal uterine bleeding not associated with either organic disease of the uterus or specific extrauterine causes of abnormal bleeding.

Anovulatory cycles (noncycling disorders) represent the most common form of dysfunctional uterine bleeding during adolescence and the climacteric. In the reproductive years they represent a significant cause of infertility. A single anovulatory cycle may occur sporadically in the majority of women and cannot be distinguished from normal proliferative phase endometrium in endometrial brushing preparations. It can only be recognized by finding a proliferative phase endometrium at a time of the cycle when a secretory pattern would be expected (see Chapter 2). After several consecutive anovulatory cycles have occurred (eg, in women with polycystic ovaries), the endometrium may reveal simple endometrial hyperplasia or even more significant endometrial hyperplasia (see Chapter 4). Clinical possibilities of anovulatory disturbances include nonfunctioning ovaries, deficient or prolonged follicular stimulation by a central or ovarian defect, and polycystic ovary. During the reproductive period, the polycystic ovary syndrome is the most important cause of anovulation. In endometrial brushing preparations from patients with anovulatory cycles, all resting or proliferative stages from atrophy to hyperplasia of the endometrium may be found.

The secretory phase defects (abnormally cycling disorders) are seen in endometria that demonstrate the effects of either inadequate or excessive progestational stimulation, and are usually associated with infertility. The deficient secretory phase may be either dissociated or coordinated.

In the deficient secretory phase with dissociated delay, the endometrium shows a variation in the development of glands and stroma (glandular stromal dyssynchrony) from region to region, and a dissociation of development between glands and their surrounding stroma. In endometrial brushing preparations, proliferative phase and secretory phase endometria coexist, secretory patterns at different stages of development are seen, or glands and stroma are dyssynchronous (see Chapter 2). Clinical possibilities of deficient secretory phase with dissociated delay include ovarian insufficiency caused by an ovarian or central defect, such as inadequate luteinization and insufficient progesterone synthesis of granulosa cells; suppression of progesterone release by hyperprolactinemia;

focal endometrial progesterone receptor defects; and irregular secretion caused by a climacteric disturbance in corpus luteum function.

In the deficient secretory phase with coordinated delay, morphologically normal secretory phase endometrium exhibits a developmental delay of 3 days or more. For instance, an endometrial brushing preparation procured on the 27th day of a menstrual cycle shows glands and stroma identical with those during the early secretory phase (see Chapter 2). Clinical possibilities of deficient secretory phase with coordinated delay include a central defect with inadequate stimulation of granulosa cells, an ovarian defect with impaired follicular development, and a diffuse defect of endometrial progesterone receptor.

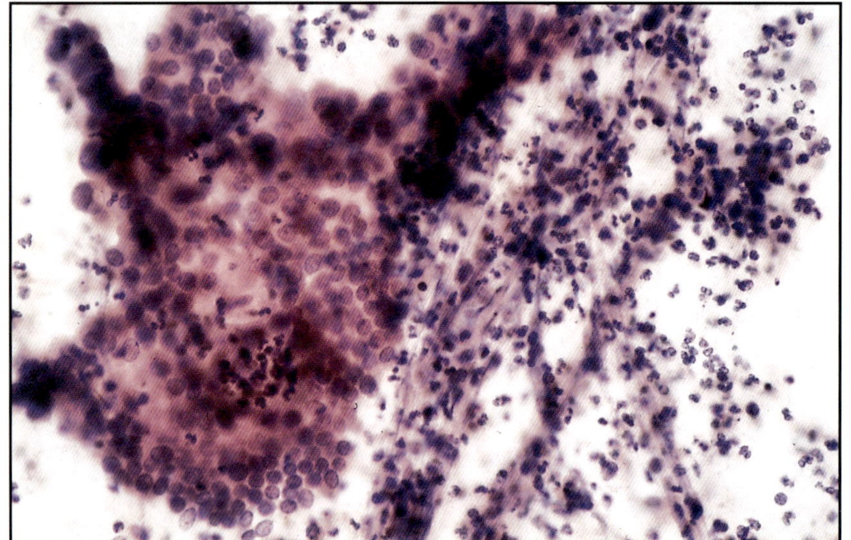

Image 3.1
Acute endometritis. There are abundant neutrophils intermixed with sheets of glandular cells. Endometrial brushing (Papanicolaou, 200X).

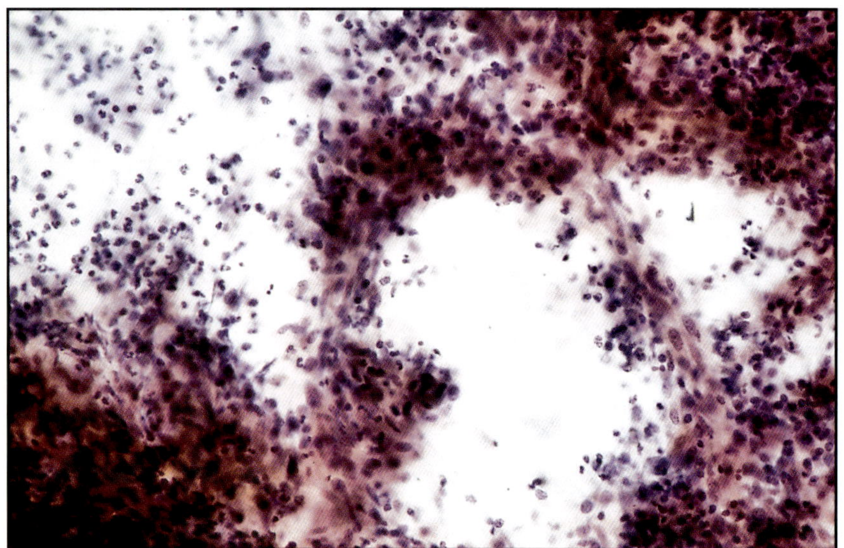

Image 3.2
Acute endometritis. There are abundant neutrophils intermixed with groupings of stromal cells. Endometrial brushing (Papanicolaou, 200X).

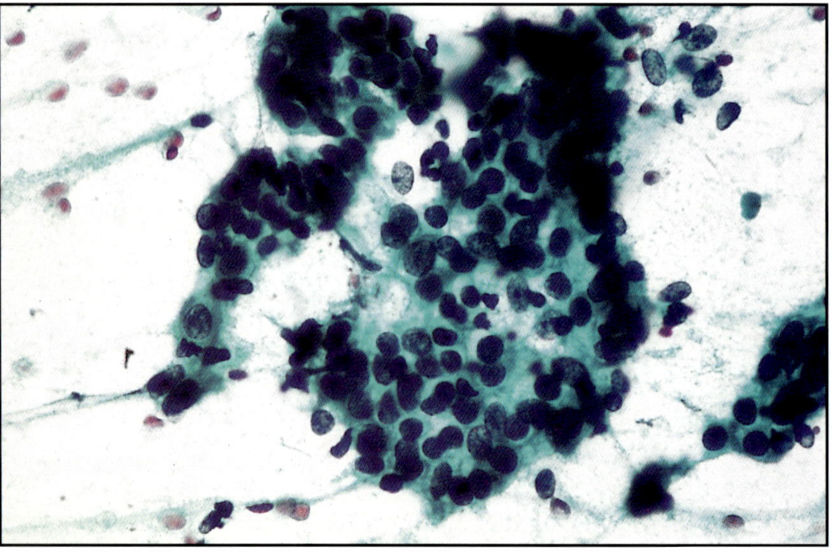

Image 3.3
Chronic endometritis. There is an admixture of glandular cells and chronic inflammatory cells including lymphocytes, plasma cells, and macrophages. The glandular cells show nuclear atypia. Endometrial brushing (Papanicolaou, 400X).

Image 3.4
Chronic endometritis. There is an admixture of stromal cells and chronic inflammatory cells including lymphocytes, plasma cells, and macrophages. Endometrial brushing (Papanicolaou, 400X).

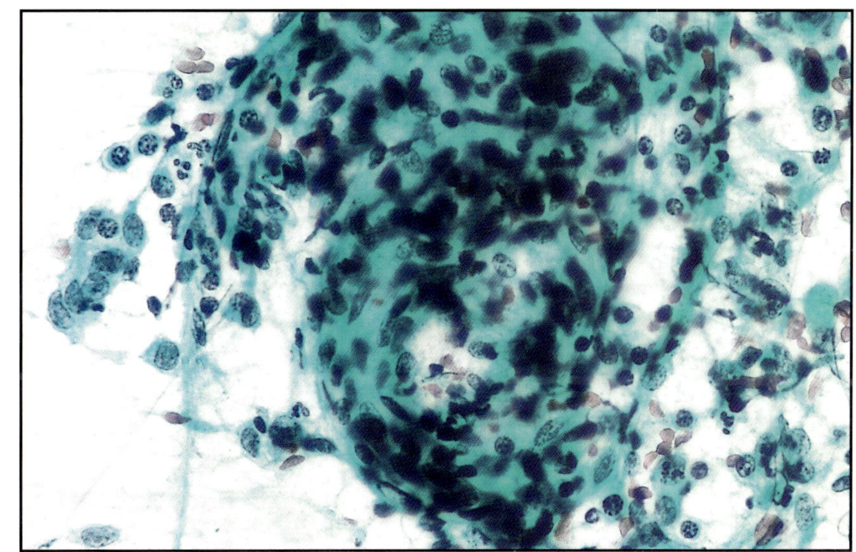

Image 3.5
Chronic endometritis. Numerous chronic inflammatory cells, including lymphocytes, plasma cells, and macrophages, are present. Occasional neutrophils are also noted. Endometrial brushing (Papanicolaou, 800X).

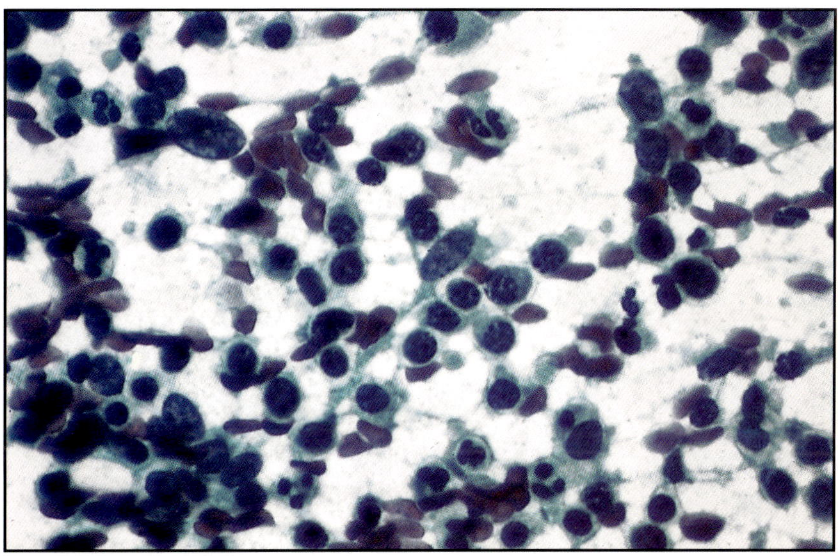

Image 3.6
Chronic endometritis. There is a heavy infiltrate of lymphocytes and plasma cells in the endometrium. Histologic section (H&E, 200X).

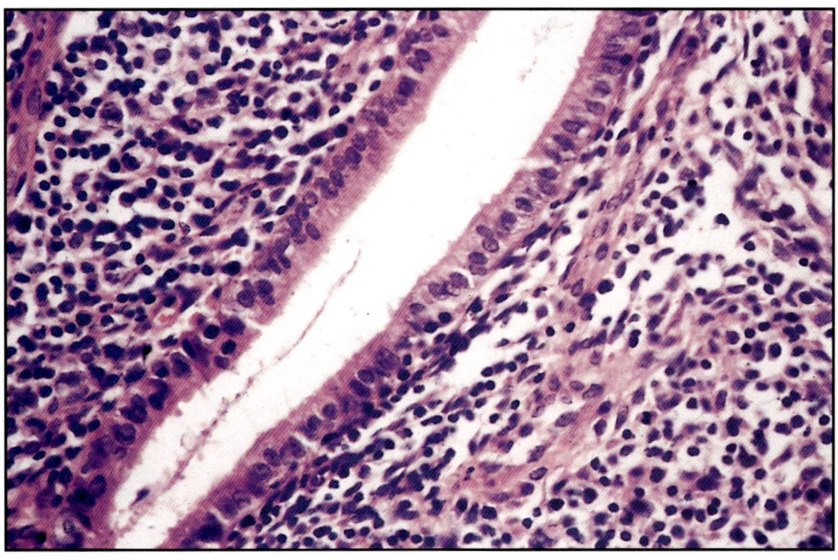

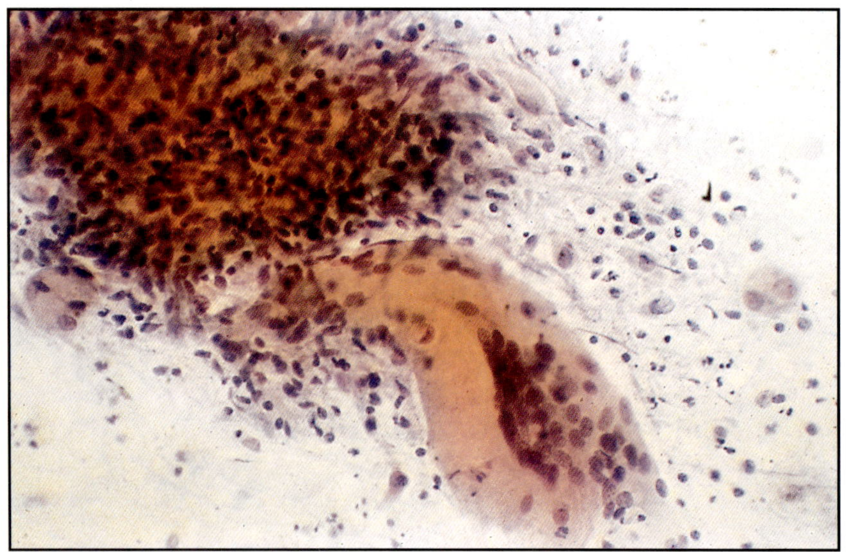

Image 3.7
Granulomatous endometritis (endometrial tuberculosis). There are abundant acute and chronic inflammatory cells intermingled with epithelioid cells, fibroblasts, and giant, multinucleated histiocytes. Endometrial brushing (Papanicolaou, 100X).

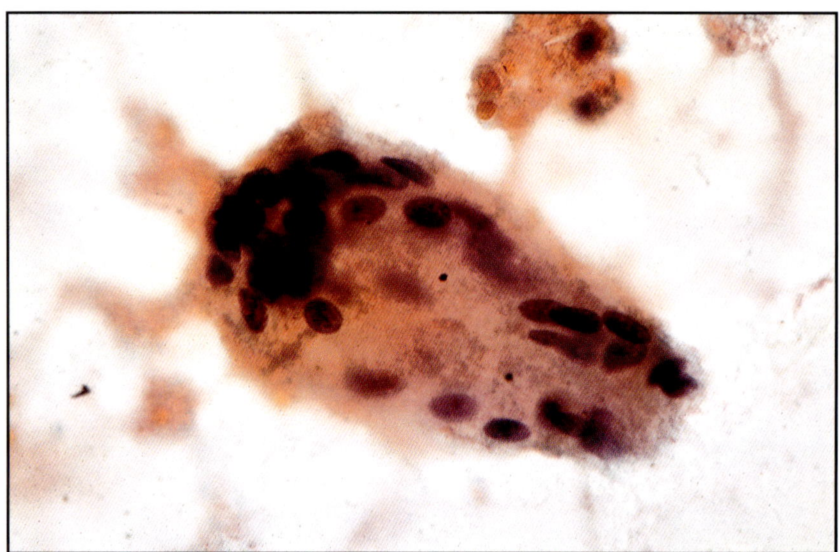

Image 3.8
Granulomatous endometritis (endometrial tuberculosis). A giant, multinucleated, Langhans-type histiocyte contains many peripherally located nuclei. Endometrial brushing (Papanicolaou, 400X).

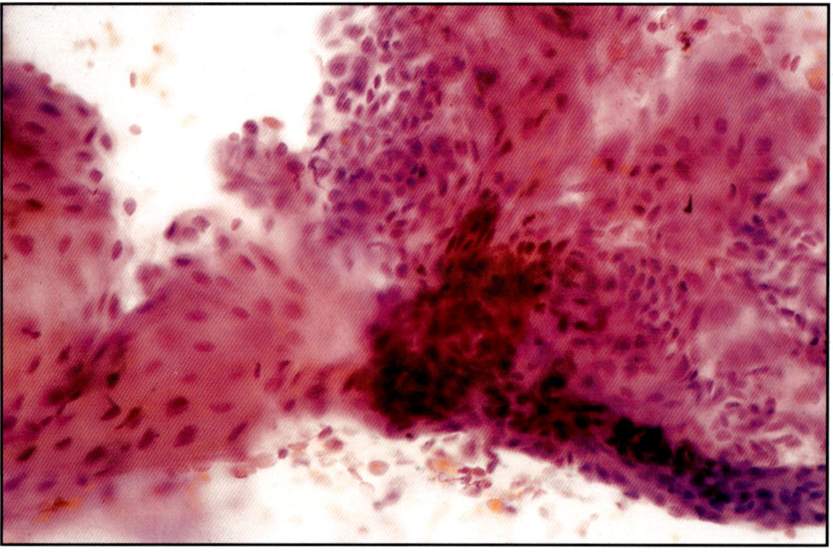

Image 3.9
Squamous metaplasia of the endometrium. Sheets of metaplastic squamous cells are in continuity with sheets of glandular cells. Endometrial brushing (Papanicolaou, 200X).

Image 3.10
Squamous metaplasis of the endometrium. Nonkeratinizing squamous
cells in berry-like aggregates are present
in the superficial layer of the endometrium. Histologic section (H&E,
100X).

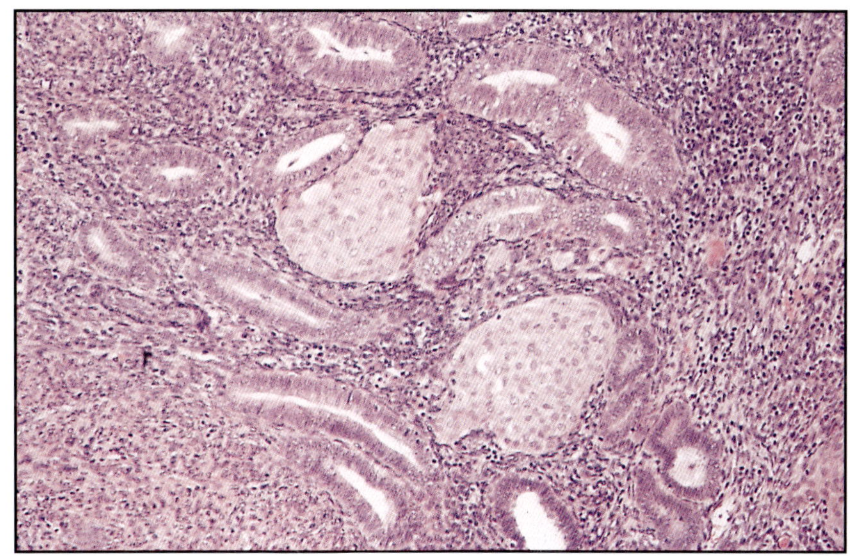

Image 3.11
Irradiation changes of the endometrium.
A few highly atypical cells that have
gigantic nuclei with coarsely granular
chromatin and an abundance of cytoplasm intermingle with some smaller,
benign-looking cells of stromal origin.
Endometrial brushing (Papanicolaou,
400X).

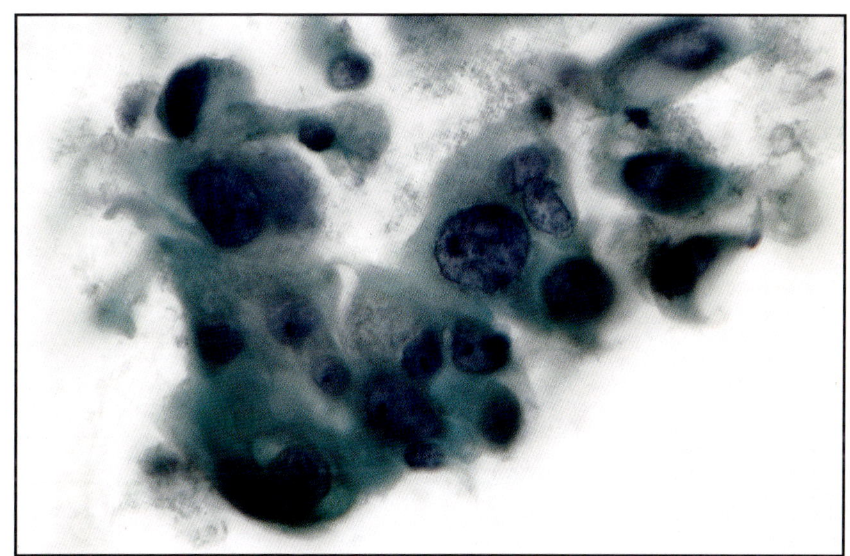

Image 3.12
Irradiation changes of the endometrium. A loose grouping of highly atypical
spindle cells with enlarged, pleomorphic, hyperchromatic or pyknotic
nuclei mimics a sarcoma. Endometrial
brushing (Papanicolaou, 400X).

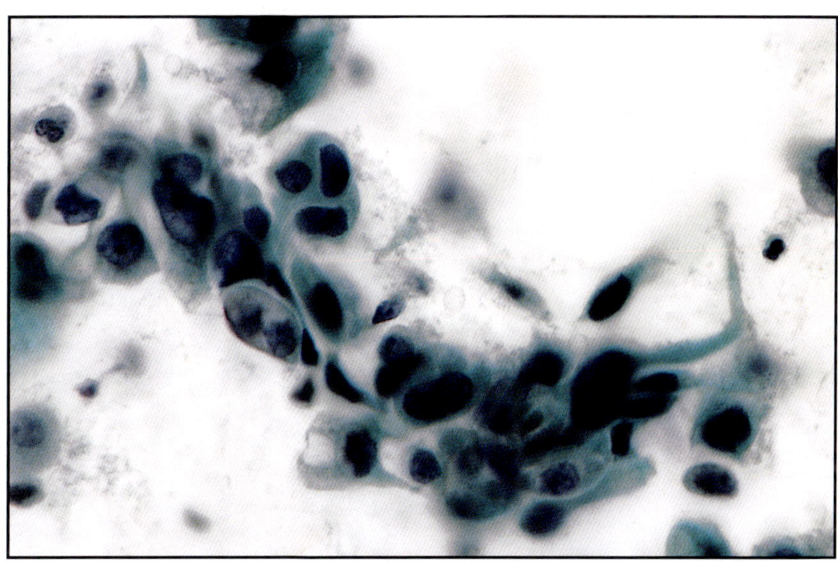

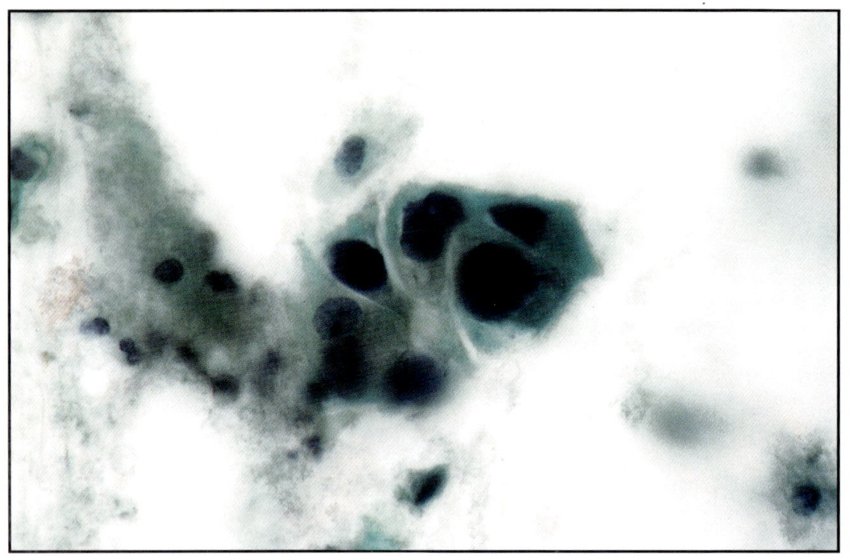

Image 3.13
Irradiation changes of the endometrium. A few highly atypical cells have large, pyknotic nuclei and a small to moderate amount of well-defined, dense cytoplasm, and mimic a squamous cell carcinoma. Endometrial brushing (Papanicolaou, 400X).

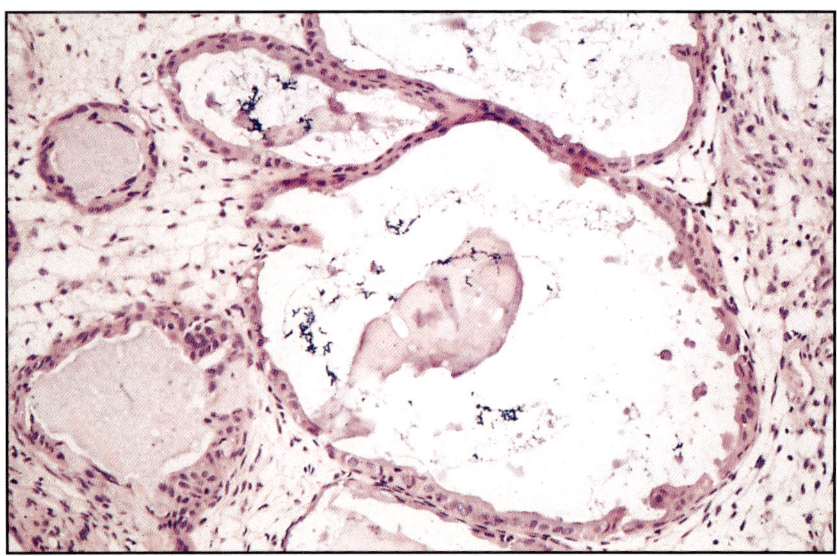

Image 3.14
Irradiation changes of the endometrium. The stroma of the endometrium undergoes cystic degeneration after radiotherapy for an endometrial adenocarcinoma. Some of the cysts are lined by metaplastic squamoid cells. Histologic section (H&E, 100X).

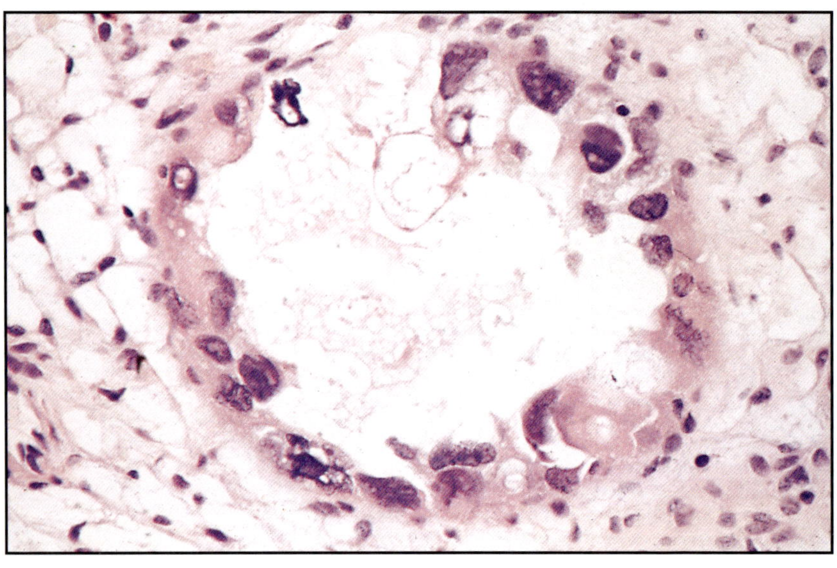

Image 3.15
Irradiation changes of the endometrium. Some of the cysts in the stroma are lined by large, bizarre cells with pleomorphic, hyperchromatic or pyknotic nuclei, resembling atypical cells shown in Images 3.12 and 3.13. Histologic section (H&E, 200X).

Image 3.16
Leiomyoma of the uterus. A bundle of smooth muscle cells with ovoid or blunt-ended elongated nuclei and abundant, ill-defined cytoplasm give a syncytial appearance. Note that the neoplastic cells from this tumor do not show any cytomorphologic difference from smooth muscle cells of the myometrium (see Image 2.34). Endometrial brushing (Papanicolaou, 400X).

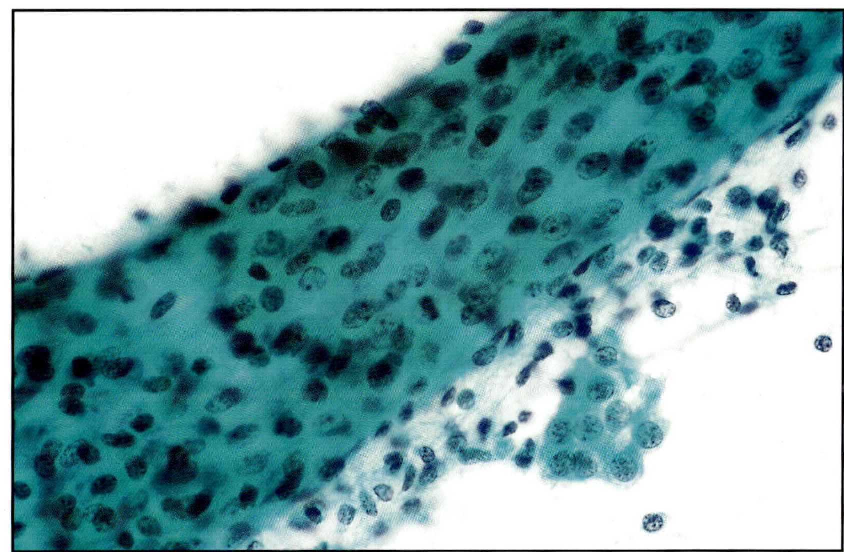

Image 3.17
Leiomyoma of the uterus. The tumors are formed by interlacing bundles of smooth muscle cells separated by well-vascularized connective tissue (not shown in this picture). Histologic section (H&E, 100X).

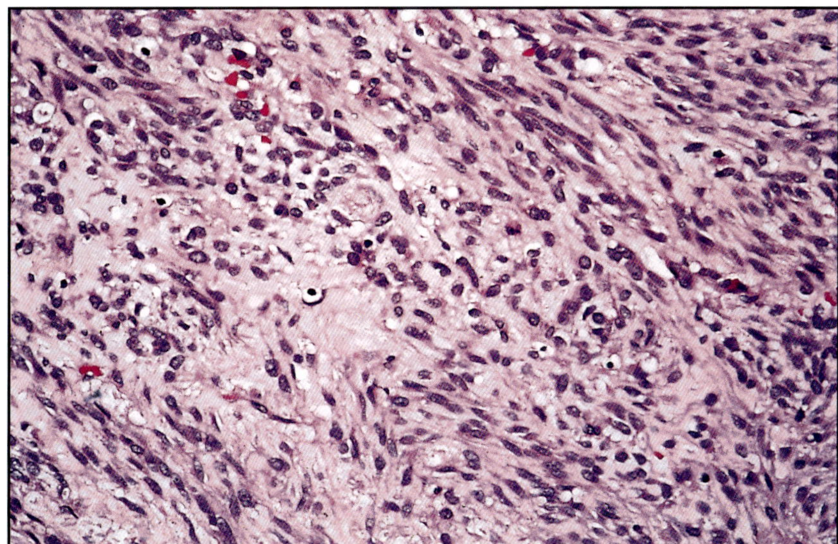

References

1. Bomze EJ, Friedman NB: Squamous metaplasia and adenoacanthosis of the endometrium. *Obstet Gynecol* 30:619–625, 1967.

2. Cadena D, Cavanzo FJ, Leone CL, et al: Chronic endometritis: A comparative clinicopathologic study. *Obstet Gynecol* 41:733–738, 1973.

3. Cassell GH, Cole BL: Mycoplasmas as agents of human disease. *N Engl J Med* 304:80, 1981.

4. Crum CP, Richart RM, Fenoglio CM: Adenoacanthosis of the endometrium: A clinicopathologic study in premenopausal women. *Am J Surg Pathol* 5:15–20, 1981.

5. Dutra FR: Intraglandular morules of the endometrium. *Am J Clin Pathol* 31:60–65, 1959.

6. Friberg J: Mycoplasmas and ureaplasmas in infertility and abortion. *Fertil Steril* 33:351–359, 1980.

7. Israel SL, Roitman HB, Clancy E: Infrequency of unsuspected endometrial tuberculosis: Histologic and bacteriologic study. *JAMA* 183:63–65, 1963.

8. Koss LG: *Diagnostic Cytology and Its Histologic Bases.* 4th ed. Philadelphia, PA, JB Lippincott Co, 1992, pp 535–587.

9. Paavonen J, Kiviat N, Brunham RC, et al: Prevalence and manifestations of endometritis among women with cervicitis. *Am J Obstet Gynecol* 152:280–286, 1985.

10. Rotterdam H: Chronic endometritis: A clinicopathologic study. *Pathol Annu* 13:209–231, 1978.

11. Whiteley PF, Hamlett JD: Pyometra: A reappraisal. *Am J Obstet Gynecol* 109:108–112, 1971.

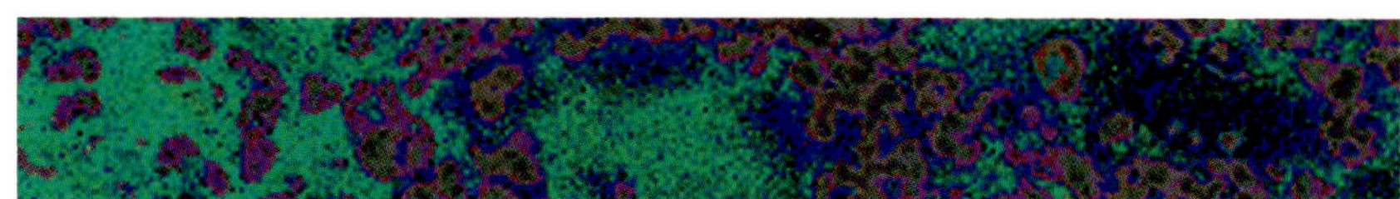

CHAPTER FOUR

Endometrial Hyperplasia

Abnormal endometrial proliferations form a morphologic continuum ranging from focal glandular crowding through various degrees of hyperplasia to carcinoma. Endometrial hyperplasia denotes an overgrowth of the endometrium that involves both glandular and stromal elements. The hyperplasia may be focal or diffuse. It may have a unicentric focus or multicentric foci of origin in the endometrium. It may be manifested in the surface epithelium or the underlying glandular epithelium. It is usually associated with an endometrium showing unopposed estrogen effect, as encountered in an anovulatory cycle, which can be recognized by finding a proliferative endometrium at a time of the cycle when a secretory pattern would be expected. Most commonly, the prolonged unremitting estrogen stimulation results in endometrial hyperplasia. To identify a focal lesion of endometrial hyperplasia, the sampling device must be able to procure samples from the entire surface of the endometrium. It is not uncommon that a random endometrial biopsy misses foci of endometrial hyperplasia.

Relationship to Endometrial Adenocarcinoma

The relationship between endometrial hyperplasia and adenocarcinoma has been debated.[14,16] Now it is clear that many cases of endometrial adenocarcinoma are preceded by endometrial hyperplasia, especially in young women. In general, the more severe the hyperplasia, the more likely it is to be followed by adenocarcinoma.[15] It is also true that relatively few patients with endometrial hyperplasia will subsequently develop adenocarcinoma, and, therefore, the mere presence of endometrial hyperplasia does not warrant hysterectomy.[15] The efficacy of hormonal therapy in controlling most cases of endometrial hyperplasia and in avoiding hysterectomy in surgically high-risk postmenopausal patients has been demonstrated repeatedly.[15] Close follow-up of treated and untreated patients with endometrial hyperplasia by periodic assessment with the IUMC Endometrial Sampler (see Chapter 1) ideally suits this purpose.

In the series reported by McBride,[12] less than 0.4% of 544 premenopausal women with cystic hyperplasia for periods ranging up to 24 years developed adenocarcinoma. Chamlian and Taylor[2] studied a long-term follow-up of 97 young women with more severe endometrial hyperplasia (adenomatous or atypical), of which 14% subsequently developed endometrial adenocarcinoma. A similar result was reported by Gusberg and Kaplan.[6]

Kurman et al[9] have demonstrated that the degree of cytologic atypia is the most useful criterion for predicting the likelihood of progression to adenocarcinoma. They reported progression to carcinoma in only 1% of patients with simple hyperplasia and in 3% of patients with complex hyperplasia.[9] In contrast, 8% of patients with simple atypical hyperplasia and 29% of patients with complex atypical hyperplasia progressed to carcinoma.[9] They concluded that the degree of cytologic atypia is more important than architectural alterations, as seen on tissue sections, to the development of endometrial adenocarcinoma.[9] The presence of cellular atypia and glandular complexity and crowding appears to place the patient at greater risk. The mean duration of progression of hyperplasia without cellular atypia to carcinoma is nearly 10 years, and it takes a mean of 4 years to progress from atypical hyperplasia to clinically evident carcinoma. This provides ample time for early detection with an annual surveillance program using cytologic techniques. In fact, in endometrial cytologic preparations procured by the IUMC Endometrial Sampler, various degrees of cellular atypia in endometrial hyperplasia can be clearly appreciated.

Histology of Endometrial Hyperplasia

Endometrial hyperplasias may be composed of various degrees of packed complex glands that may display cytologic atypia. These hyperplastic lesions of the endometrium comprise a gray area in the spectrum and provide the greatest difficulty in interpretation, since some well-differentiated adenocarcinomas of the endometrium lack significant atypia and some hyperplasias show atypia to a marked degree.[15] Much confusion about the premalignant significance of endometrial hyperplasia results from the absence of a uniformly accepted terminology for these hyperplastic lesions. In the 1970s, endometrial hyperplasia was classified into three types: cystic hyperplasia, adenomatous hyperplasia, and atypical hyperplasia.[18,19] This classification is essentially based on architectural patterns that cannot be appreciated in cytologic preparations. However, the basic pathology of endometrial hyperplasia includes two kinds of

Beutler et al[1]	Gore and Hertig[5]	Vellios[19]	Hendrickson and Kempson[7]	Rosai[15]
Cystic proliferation	Cystic hyperplasia	Cystic hyperplasia	Hyperplasia without atypia/ with mild atypia	Mild hyperplasia
Glandular hyperplasia	Adenomatous hyperplasia	Adenomatous hyperplasia	Hyperplasia with moderate atypia	Moderate hyperplasia
Glandular hyperplasia with atypical epithelial proliferation	Anaplasia; carcinoma in-situ	Atypical hyperplasia; carcinoma in-situ	Hyperplasia with severe atypia	Severe hyperplasia

Cellular changes are more important than architectural changes in the development of endometrial carcinoma

atypical changes: (1) architectural changes, eg, cystic dilation, an increase in number of glands, and back to back arrangements of glands; and (2) cellular changes, eg, various degrees of cellular atypia of glandular epithelial cells.[11] Most authors agree that cellular changes are more important than architectural changes in relation to the development of endometrial carcinoma.[9] In the 1980s, some authors proposed classifications of endometrial hyperplasia on the basis of cellular atypia, which can be clearly demonstrated in cytologic preparations.[7] In fact, cellular atypia can be better appreciated in cytologic preparations than on tissue sections. A comparison of some important classifications of endometrial hyperplasia is presented in Table 4.1.

In recent years, the International Society of Gynecological Pathologists has proposed a new classification of endometrial hyperplasia, namely, *simple*, *complex* (adenomatous without atypia), and *atypical* (complex with atypia). Rosai, in his surgical pathology textbook,[15] classified endometrial hyperplasia into three grades: *mild* (simple), *moderate* (adenomatous), and *severe* (atypical). He disregarded the presence or absence of cystic changes, which are thought to be a secondary feature of the process and can be found in the absence of endometrial hyperplasia.[15] He also pointed out that there is rough inverse relationship between the presence and prominence of the cystic changes and the degree of glandular hyperplasia.[15]

Gore and Hertig[5] have designated a histologic pattern characterized by endometrial glands composed of large cells with abundant eosinophilic cytoplasm as carcinoma in situ. Since their assumption that this change inevitably progresses to invasive adenocarcinoma has never been proven and this change has, on occasion, been reversed by hormone manipulations, many authors prefer to regard this and similar histologic patterns as morphologic variants of atypical hyperplasia.[1,15]

Cystic Hyperplasia

Cystic hyperplasia (simple or mild hyperplasia) is the most common form of endometrial hyperplasia. On the histologic sections of cystic hyperplasia there is an overgrowth of endometrial tissue consisting of normal-sized and dilated glands separated by hyperplastic stroma. The glands are lined by tall columnar or cuboidal epithelium showing some degree of mitotic activity and mild stratification. The nuclei are usually not enlarged and the nucleoli are inconspicuous (Images 4.1 and 4.2). There is abundant stroma separating the dilated glands. The stromal cells may be increased in size with frequent mitoses. The mild stratification of columnar epithelial cells seen in this form of hyperplasia distinguishes it from cystic (senile) atrophy, since the latter are lined by a single layer of flattened or low cuboidal epithelium.

Adenomatous Hyperplasia

Microscopically, there are outpouchings and infoldings of the pro-liferating endometrial glands forming bud-like projections in cases of adenomatous hyperplasia (complex or moderate hyperplasia). These projections may become pinched off to form small nests of closely packed glands. These glands, however, have the same staining qualities as the proliferative phase endometrium. They are lined by tall columnar cells with uniform ovoid nuclei, and stratification of the epithelial cells is inconspicuous. Numerous mitotic figures are present in both the stroma and glands (Image 4.3).

Atypical Hyperplasia

Atypical hyperplasia (complex hyperplasia with atypia, or severe hyperplasia) is usually characterized by a greatly increased number of large glands, which are closely related and separated by very little inter-vening stroma. Intraglandular tufting of the epithelium may be present, but no bridging is seen. The glandular epithelial cells are enlarged and show various degrees of cellular atypia. The amount of cytoplasm is variable. The nuclei are also enlarged and appear round or ovoid with frequent conspicuous nucleoli and dense chromatin. Stratification of the epithelial cells is evident and the nuclei have an altered polarity. Numerous mitotic figures are often noted (Image 4.4).

Stromal hyperplasia usually coexists with glandular hyperplasia. In the mild and moderate endometrial hyperplasias, the stromal cells are more densely packed than in proliferative phase endometrium. The stromal cells retain their spindle shape and have enlarged, plump nuclei and ill-defined cytoplasm. Mitotic activity in endometrial stromal cells is increased but variable. Cytologic atypia is rarely noted. In the severe endometrial hyperplasia, the stromal cells are spindle-shaped and become compressed by the glandular proliferation. In addition to densely packed stromal cells, clusters of stromal foam cells occur in the stroma of 30% of the mild or moderate endometrial hyperplasia and in 53% of the severe endometrial hyperplasia.[3]

Cytology of Endometrial Hyperplasia

Relevant studies of the cellular changes in endometrial hyperplasia are limited. It is often very difficult or impossible to diagnose endometrial

Cytomorphologically, endometrial hyperplasia can be classified into three grades: mild, moderate, and severe

hyperplasia on the basis of cervicovaginal smears, because they depend solely on spontaneously desquamated endometrial cells that are usually scant, inadequately preserved, and inconstant in their occurrence. However, samples collected directly from the endometrial cavity contain a large concentration of cells and provide plenty of material for cytomorphologic study. In recent years, Kurman et al[9] classified endometrial hyperplasia according to the degree of nuclear abnormality. Based on their observation, endometrial carcinoma developed in only 2 (1.6%) of 122 patients without significant cytologic atypia and in 11 (23%) of 48 patients with "atypical" glandular epithelia. They reported that the mean duration of progression of endometrial hyperplasia without cellular atypia to carcinoma is nearly 10 years, and it takes a mean of 4 years to progress from atypical hyperplasia with cellular atypia to clinically evident carcinoma. This provides ample time for early detection of the precursors of endometrial adenocarcinoma or small occult adenocarcinoma by cytologic techniques. Cytomorphologically, endometrial hyperplasia can be classified into three grades on the basis of cytologic atypia, namely, mild, moderate, and severe, which correspond to Rosai's classification of endometrial hyperplasia.[15] The cytologic features of various degrees of endometrial hyperplasia are summarized below.

Mild Endometrial Hyperplasia

In endometrial brushing preparations, the hyperplastic glandular cells occur in sheet arrangements with apparent nuclear crowding. The average nuclear size is slightly increased (as compared to normal proliferative glandular cells), and the nuclei are round or ovoid. They are relatively uniform and regular, but slight variation in nuclear size is seen in some groups of glandular cells. The nuclear outlines are very close to each other, and nuclear overlapping is present. Overcrowding of nuclei and slightly disorganized cellular arrangements may be encountered in some cohesive groupings of glandular cells. The chromatin pattern is finely granular or slightly coarse. Small nucleoli are seen in some of the glandular cells (Images 4.5–4.8). The stromal cells with ill-defined cytoplasm are often more densely packed than in proliferative phase endometrium. Their nuclei are slightly enlarged and appear plump. Mitotic activity in glandular and stromal cells is variable and is increased in some cases. Any endometrial preparations from postmenopausal women showing mitotic activity in endometrial cells should be carefully examined and investigated.

Moderate Endometrial Hyperplasia

In endometrial brushing preparations, the hyperplastic glandular cells occur in flat sheets with apparent nuclear crowding and overlapping. Their nuclei are enlarged and show variations in nuclear size and shape, but most of them are still round or ovoid. The cytoplasm is scant and ill-defined. The chromatin is slightly coarsely granular, and conspicuous nucleoli are present in some of the glandular cells. The disorganized cellular arrangements and the overcrowding of nuclei may be encountered in some cohesive groupings of glandular cells (Images 4.9–4.12). The stromal cells are densely packed. These cells retain their spindle shape and have

Increase in average nuclear size

Variations in nuclear size and shape

Sheet arrangements with nuclear overlapping and crowding

Presence of mitotic figures in a postmenopausal woman

Slightly coarsely granular chromatin pattern

Presence of small or prominent nucleoli in some cells

Presence of stromal foam cells

---

enlarged, plump nuclei and ill-defined cytoplasm. Clusters of stromal foam cells may be observed. Mitotic activity in both glandular and stromal cells is increased and the mitotic figures are easy to find.

Severe Endometrial Hyperplasia

In endometrial brushing preparation, the hyperplastic glandular cells occur in flat sheets, or in three-dimensional, cohesive groupings, with relatively regular cellular arrangements in some groups and disorganized cellular arrangements in other groups. Their nuclei are significantly enlarged and show marked variations in nuclear size and shape. Some of them are irregularly shaped. Small or prominent nucleoli may be seen in some cells. In some cases the cytoplasm is relatively scant, and in other cases the cytoplasm appears abundant but ill-defined. The chromatin is slightly coarse or rarely coarsely granular, and the nuclei appear hyperchromatic in some cells (Images 4.13–4.16). The stromal cells are relatively scant as compared with the number of glandular cells seen in the endometrial brushing preparation. They retain their spindle shape with plump nuclei and scant, ill-defined cytoplasm. Clusters of stromal foam cells may be seen (Image 4.17). Mitotic figures are usually easy to find.

In histologic diagnosis of endometrial lesions, a great deal of experience is needed to distinguish an extreme case of severe endometrial hyperplasia from a well-differentiated adenocarcinoma, largely because of the fact that endometrial hyperplasia and carcinoma represent different points in a disease continuum at the light microscopic, ultrastructural, immunocytochemical, and biochemical levels.[4,17] Microscopic features favoring carcinoma include marked pleomorphism with loss of polarity, complex ramification of disorderly arranged glands, extensive papillary formations, confluent glandular pattern with a solid or cribriform appearance, presence of intraglandular cellular bridges devoid of stromal support, and desmoplastic (fibroblastic) stroma.[8,10,13] However, histologic patterns seen on tissue sections are not present in cytologic preparations. In cytologic diagnosis, the criteria used to distinguish severe endometrial hyperplasia from a well-differentiated adenocarcinoma are different. This is discussed in Chapter 5. The cytologic criteria used for diagnosing mild or moderate endometrial hyperplasia are summarized in Table 4.2.

The cytologic diagnosis of endometrial hyperplasia should be always based on overall cytologic findings, because there is some cytomorphologic overlapping among proliferative phase endometrium, endometrial

The cytologic diagnosis of endometrial hyperplasia should be always based on overall cytologic findings

hyperplasia, and well-differentiated adenocarcinoma. It is possible to diagnose endometrial hyperplasia in postmenopausal women on cytologic grounds, but it can be difficult or impossible to diagnose cytomorphologically mild or moderate endometrial hyperplasia in premenopausal women. In this cytologic classification of endometrial hyperplasia, only cases showing nuclear atypia are included. The weakly proliferative endometrium (seen in perimenopausal or postmenopausal women whose endometria are weakly supported by low levels of endogenous or exogenous estrogen) and disordered proliferative endometrium (seen in perimenopausal women with sporadic anovulatory cycles or those receiving estrogen therapy; see Chapter 2) are not included in this classification, unless nuclear atypia is identified.

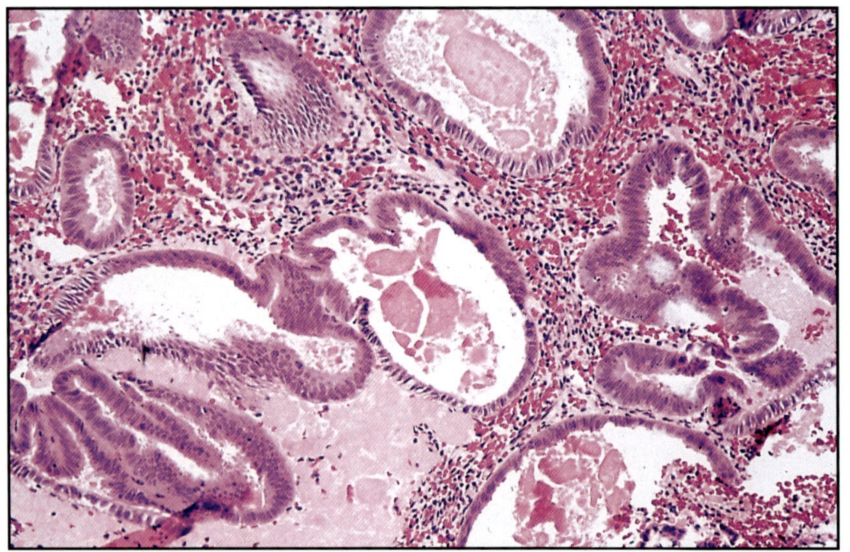

Image 4.1

Cystic hyperplasia of the endometrium. There is an overgrowth of endometrial tissue consisting of normal and dilated glands. The glands are lined by tall columnar or cuboidal epithelium. Mild stratification of columnar epithelial cells is present. Histologic section (H&E, 100X).

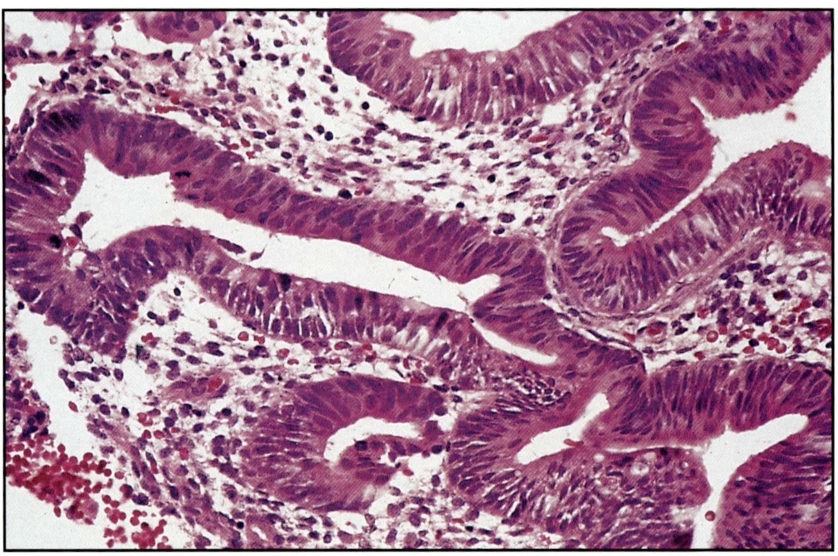

Image 4.2

Cystic hyperplasia of the endometrium. Higher-power view of cystic hyperplasia showing mild stratification of columnar epithelial cells. Occasional mitotic figures are noted. Histologic section (H&E, 200X).

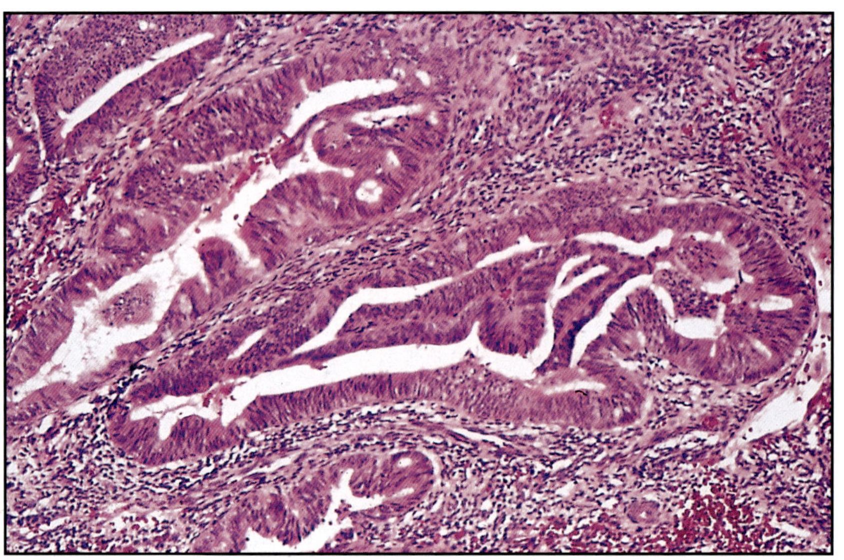

Image 4.3

Adenomatous hyperplasia of the endometrium. There are outpouchings and infoldings of the proliferating endometrial glands forming bud-like projections. These glands are lined by tall columnar cells with uniform ovoid nuclei, and stratification of the epithelial cells is present. Histologic section (H&E, 100X).

Image 4.4
Atypical hyperplasia of the endometrium. A large gland exhibits prominent intraglandular tufting of the
epithelium. The glandular epithelial
cells are enlarged and show various
degrees of cellular atypia. The enlarged
nuclei appear round or ovoid with
dense chromatin and have an altered
polarity. Histologic section (H&E,
200X).

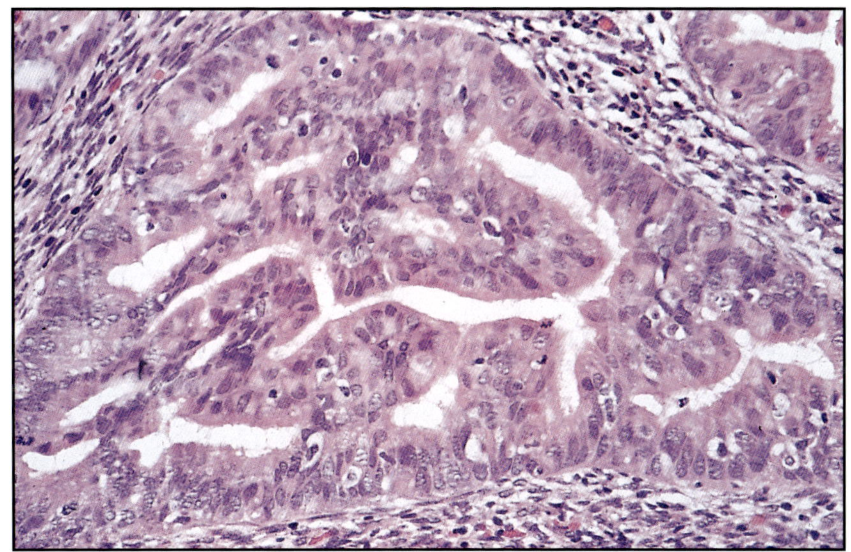

Image 4.5
Mild endometrial hyperplasia in a postmenopausal woman. The proliferating
glandular cells occur in sheet arrangements with apparent nuclear crowding
and overlapping. Their nuclei are
slightly enlarged and have frequent,
small nucleoli and slightly coarse chromatin. Occasional mitotic figures are
noted. Endometrial brushing (Papanicolaou, 400X).

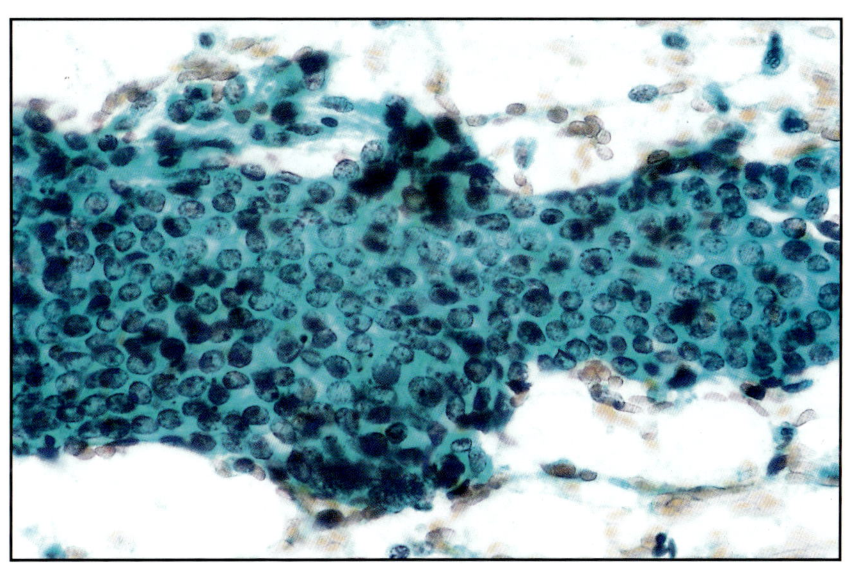

Image 4.6
Mild endometrial hyperplasia in a postmenopausal woman. The proliferating
glandular cells exhibit some variation in
nuclear size. The cellular arrangements
are slightly disorganized. Endometrial
brushing (Papanicolaou, 400X).

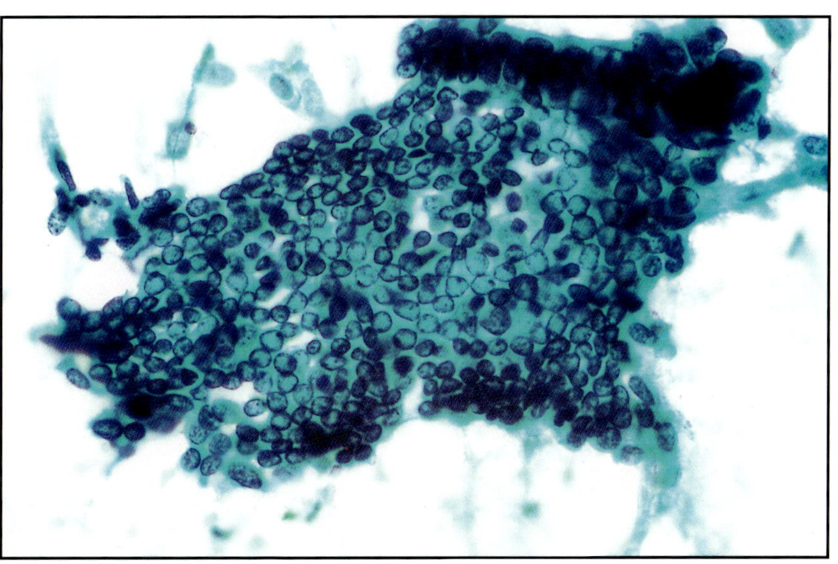

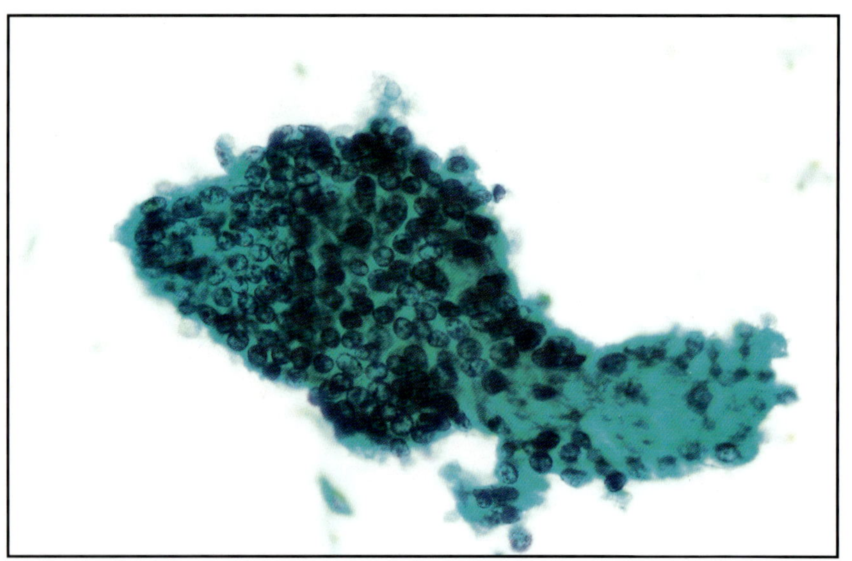

Image 4.7
Mild endometrial hyperplasia in a post-menopausal woman. The proliferating glandular cells have round or ovoid, dense nuclei and occur in a cohesive grouping. Overcrowding of the nuclei is noticed. Endometrial brushing (Papanicolaou, 400X).

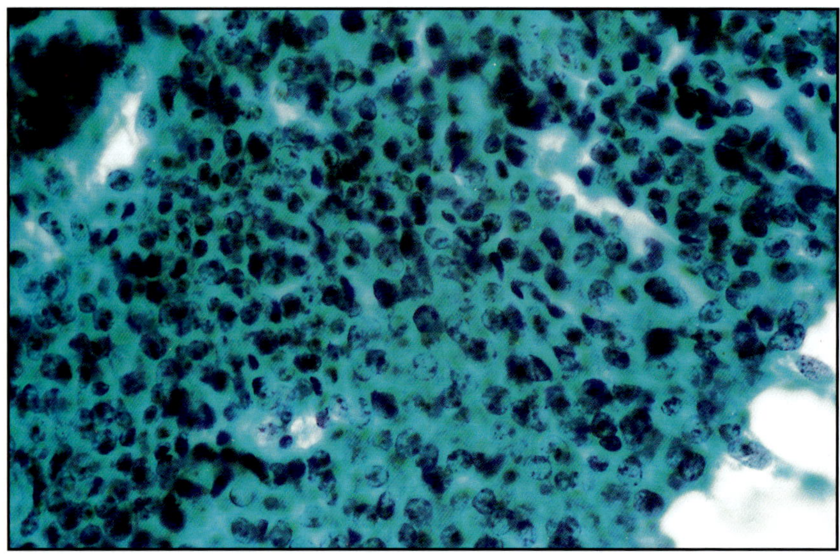

Image 4.8
Mild endometrial hyperplasia in a post-menopausal woman. Slightly disorganized sheets of epithelial cells consist of proliferating glandular cells that have dense nuclei with slightly coarse chromatin and frequent small nucleoli. Some variation in nuclear size is also noticed. Endometrial brushing (Papanicolaou, 400X).

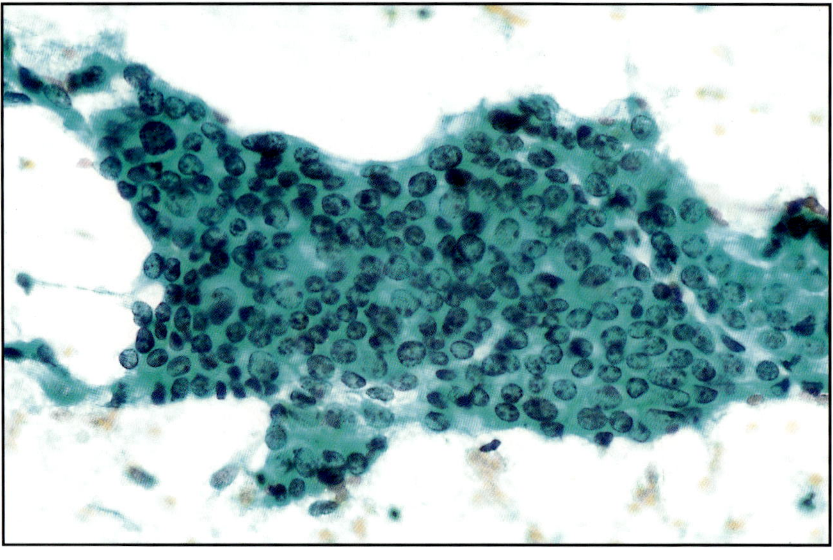

Image 4.9
Moderate endometrial hyperplasia in a postmenopausal woman. The proliferating glandular cells have enlarged nuclei with dense chromatin and frequent small nucleoli. Variation in nuclear size is evident. Endometrial brushing (Papanicolaou, 400X).

Image 4.10
Moderate endometrial hyperplasia in a
postmenopausal woman. Disorganized
sheets of glandular epithelium consist
of enlarged, crowding, proliferating
glandular cells with dense nuclei and
frequent small nucleoli. Variation in
nuclear size is also noticed. Endometrial
brushing (Papanicolaou, 400X).

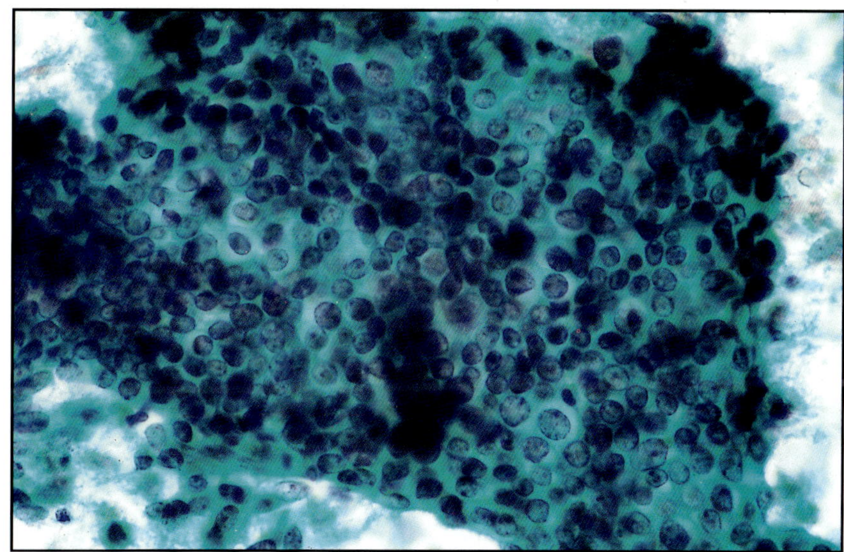

Image 4.11
Moderate endometrial hyperplasia in a
postmenopausal woman. The proliferating glandular cells have enlarged,
round or ovoid nuclei and scant, ill-
defined cytoplasm. They occur in flat
sheet arrangements with apparent
nuclear crowding and overlapping.
Endometrial brushing (Papanicolaou,
400X).

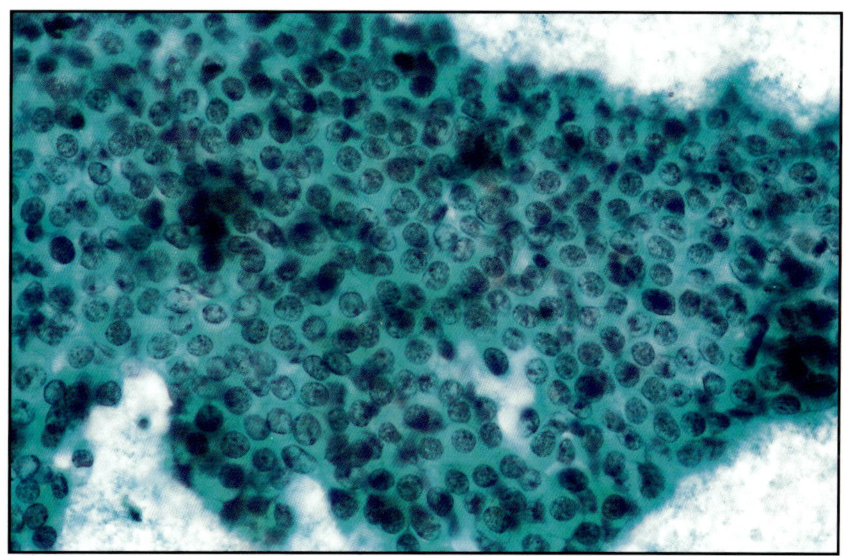

Image 4.12
Moderate endometrial hyperplasia in a
postmenopausal woman. The proliferating glandular cells have hyperchromatic, round or ovoid nuclei with
slightly coarsely granular chromatin,
and occur in a cohesive grouping.
Overcrowding of the nuclei is noticed.
Endometrial brushing (Papanicolaou,
400X).

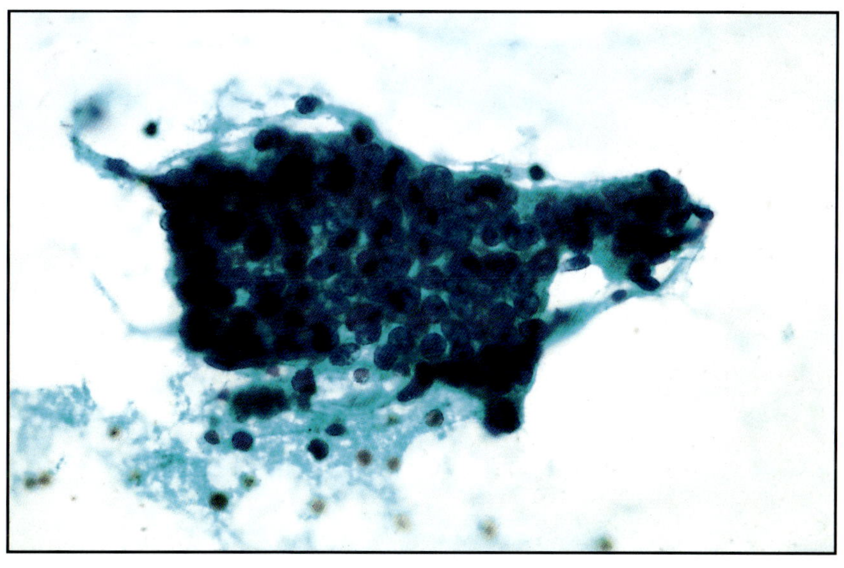

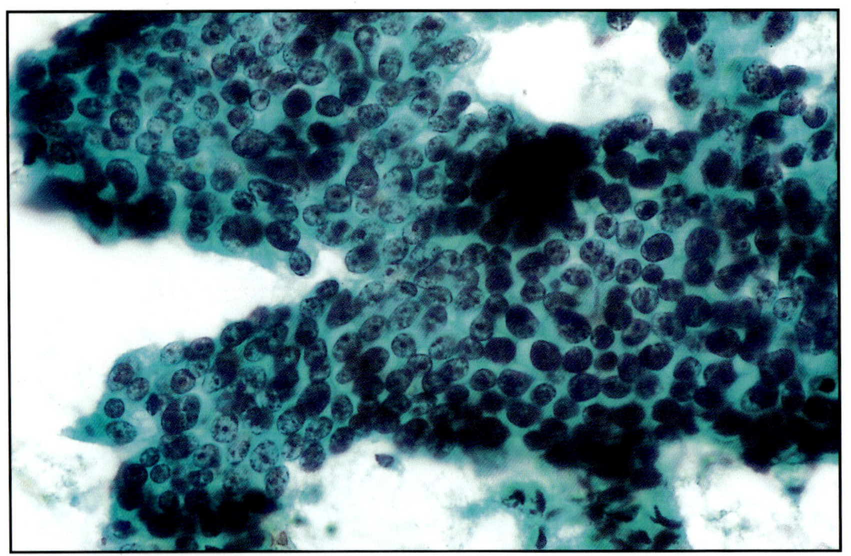

Image 4.13
Severe endometrial hyperplasia. The atypical glandular cells have relatively large nuclei with slightly coarse or coarsely granular chromatin and frequent, small or prominent nucleoli, mimicking a well-differentiated endometrial adenocarcinoma. Endometrial brushing (Papanicolaou, 400X).

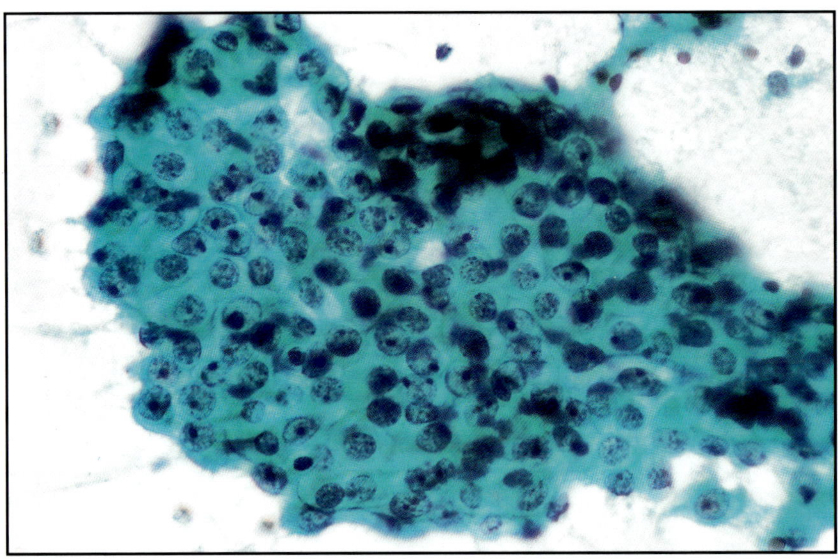

Image 4.14
Severe endometrial hyperplasia. The atypical glandular cells have large nuclei with frequent prominent nucleoli and a moderate amount to an abundance of cytoplasm, and occur in a cohesive grouping. They exhibit marked variation in nuclear size. Endometrial brushing (Papanicolaou, 400X).

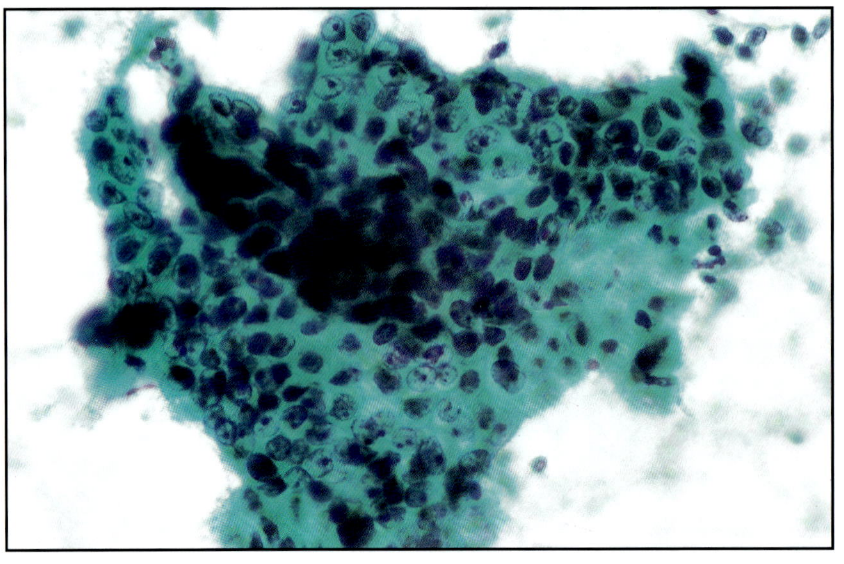

Image 4.15
Severe endometrial hyperplasia. The atypical glandular cells have relatively large, hyperchromatic nuclei with slightly coarse or coarsely granular chromatin and a small to moderate amount of ill-defined cytoplasm. They occur in a cohesive grouping with an altered polarity. Prominent nuclei are present in some cells. Endometrial brushing (Papanicolaou, 400X).

Image 4.16
Severe endometrial hyperplasia. The stromal cells have plump nuclei with fine chromatin and scant, ill-defined cytoplasm, and occur in loose or cohesive groupings. Endometrial brushing (Papanicolaou, 400X).

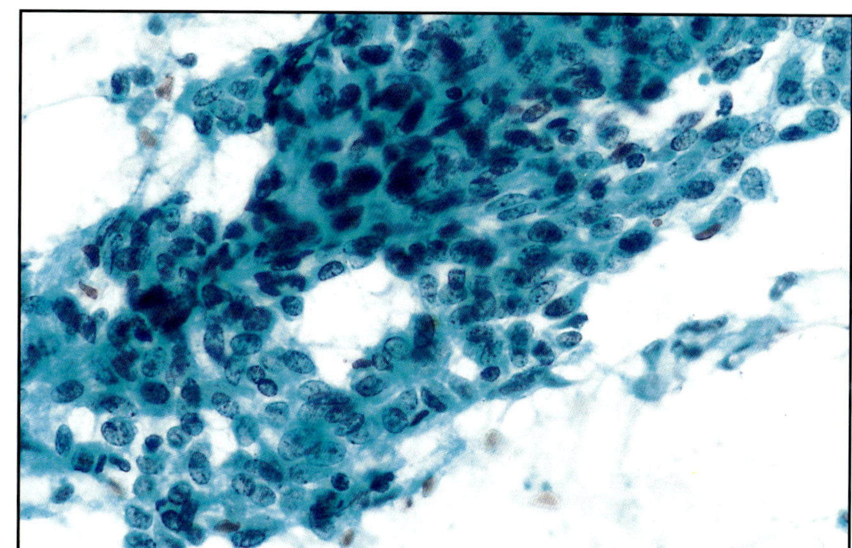

Image 4.17
Stromal foam cells in endometrial hyperplasia. The stromal foam cells have relatively large, centrally located, ovoid nuclei and an abundance of foamy cytoplasm. They occur in a cohesive grouping. These cells are morphologically identical to the stromal foam cells seen in the stroma of endometrial adenocarcinoma. Endometrial brushing (Papanicolaou, 400X).

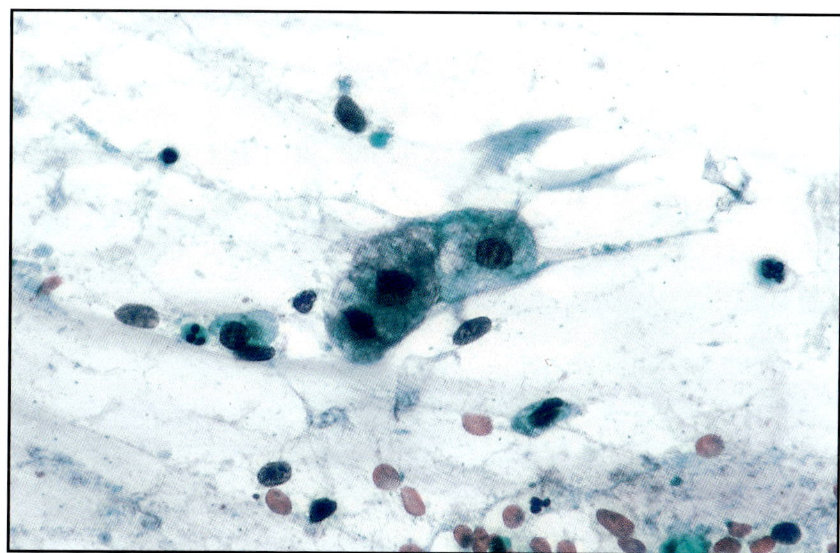

References

1. Beutler HK, Dockerty MB, Randall LM: Precancerous lesions of the endometrium. *Am J Obstet Gynecol* 86:433–443, 1963.

2. Chamlian LD, Taylor HB: Endometrial hyperplasia in young women. *Obstet Gynecol* 36:659–666, 1970.

3. Fechner RE, Bossarl MI, Spjut R: Ultrastructure of endometrial stromal foam cells. *Am J Clin Pathol* 72:628–633, 1979.

4. Fenoglio CM, Crum CP, Ferenzy A: Endometrial hyperplasia and carcinoma: Are ultrastructural, biochemical and immunocytochemical studies useful in distinguishing between them? *Pathol Res Pract* 174:256–284, 1982.

5. Gore H, Hertig AT: Carcinoma in situ of the endometrium. *Am J Obstet Gynecol* 94:135–155, 1966.

6. Gusberg SB, Kaplan AL: Precursors of corpus cancer: IV. Adenomatous hyperplasia as stage 0 carcinoma of the endometrium. *Am J Obstet Gynecol* 87:662–676, 1963.

7. Hendrickson MR, Kempson RL: Surgical pathology of the uterine corpus. In: *Major Problems in Pathology,* vol 12, Bennington JL (editor). Philadelphia, PA, WB Saunders Co, 1980, pp 285–318.

8. Hendrickson MR, Ross JC, Kempson RL: Toward the development of morphologic criteria for well-differentiated adenocarcinoma of the endometrium. *Am J Surg Pathol* 7:819–838, 1983.

9. Kurman RJ, Kaminski RF, Norris HJ: The behavior of endometrial hyperplasia: A long-term study of "untreated" hyperplasia in 170 patients. *Cancer* 56:403–412, 1985.

10. Kurman RJ, Norris HJ: Evaluation of criteria for distinguishing atypical endometrial hyperplasia from well-differentiated carcinoma. *Cancer* 49:2547–2559, 1982.

11. Kurman RJ, Norris HJ: Endometrium. In: *The Pathology of Incipient Neoplasia,* Henson DE, Albores-Saavedra J (editors). Philadelphia, PA, WB Saunders Co, 1986, pp 265–277.

12. McBride JM: Premenopausal cystic hyperplasia and endometrial carcinoma. *J Obstet Gynecol Br Emp* 66:288–296, 1959.

13. Norris HJ, Tavassoli FA, Kurman RJ: Endometrial hyperplasia and carcinoma: Diagnostic considerations. *Am J Surg Pathol* 7:839–847, 1983.

14. Rome M, Brown JB, Mason T, et al: Estrogen excretion and ovarian pathology in postmenopausal women with atypical hyperplasia, adenocarcinoma and mixed adenosquamous carcinoma of the endometrium. *Br J Obstet Gynecol* 84:88–97, 1977.

15. Rosai J: *Ackerman's Surgical Pathology.* 7th ed. St Louis, MO, CV Mosby, 1989, pp 1050–1097.

16. Scully RE: Definition of precursors in gynecologic cancer. *Cancer* 48:531–537, 1981.

17. Soderström K-O: Lectin binding to human endometrial hyperplasia and adenocarcinoma. *Int J Gynecol Pathol* 6:356–365, 1987.

18. Tavassoli F, Kraus FT: Endometrial lesions in uteri resected for atypical endometrial hyperplasia. *Am J Clin Pathol* 70:770–779, 1978.

19. Vellios F: Endometrial hyperplasia: Precursors of endometrial carcinoma. *Pathol Annu* 7:201–229, 1972.

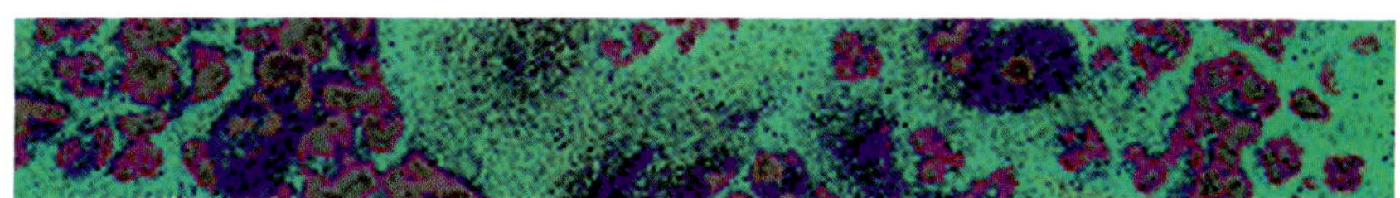

CHAPTER FIVE

Endometrial Carcinoma

Endometrial carcinoma has become the most common gynecologic malignancy in the United States, and its incidence is rising. It typically occurs in elderly patients. Patients at high risk include the diabetic, obese, hypertensive, and infertile; those with late-onset menopause[7,8,10,27,29,30]; those with failure of ovulation and dysfunctional bleeding; long-standing estrogen users[3,21]; those with severe endometrial hyperplasia; those with the Stein-Leventhal syndrome; and those with functioning granulosa cell tumors and thecomas.[23,26] Gonadal dysgenesis (Turner's syndrome) may also be associated with endometrial carcinoma, and most of these patients have received replacement estrogen therapy, usually in high dosages for prolonged periods.[14] The common denominator for many of these risk factors is excess estrogenic stimulation.[13,15]

Several studies have shown a high incidence of both endometrial carcinoma and breast carcinoma among sisters, mothers, and aunts of individuals with endometrial carcinoma, suggesting a genetic predisposition.[12,17] In particular, endometrial adenosquamous carcinoma tends to be associated with breast carcinoma.

According to some authors, there may be two different types of endometrial carcinoma: type I, a low-grade neoplasm that is estrogen related and occurs in younger, perimenopausal women; and type II, a more virulent form, unrelated to estrogenic stimulation, that occurs in older postmenopausal women.[2,5] Robboy and Bradley[22] showed that the endometrial carcinomas in estrogen users are better differentiated than those in nonestrogen users. Only 4 (12%) of 33 of the estrogen users had poorly differentiated adenocarcinoma compared with 30 (37%) of 81 of the nonusers, suggesting that the development of poorly differentiated adenocarcinoma is unrelated to the use of estrogen. These findings suggest that endometrial hyperplasia is a precursor of type I endometrial carcinoma. Endometrial carcinomas that have an unfavorable prognosis, such as clear cell carcinoma and adenosquamous carcinoma, may be unrelated to estrogen use. They occur at an older age (mean age, 66 years) and are rarely associated with endometrial hyperplasia.

Adenocarcinoma of the Endometrium

Adenocarcinoma accounts for approximately 90% of malignant tumors of the uterine corpus. It usually begins on the surface of the endometrium, and it presents in one of two macroscopic forms: localized or diffuse. Localized carcinoma consists of a round, polypoid or exophytic mass, which is friable and often shows surface ulceration. The uterine cavity is progressively encroached on by soft, easily detachable, neoplastic masses. Diffuse carcinoma extensively infiltrates the thickened and indurated mucosa. The volume of the uterus is usually increased, and the uterine cavity is filled with tumor, which may block the cervical canal and cause pyometra. Five to fifteen percent of the cases of postmenopausal bleeding are due to endometrial carcinoma.[16,19]

Histologically, endometrial adenocarcinomas can be divided into well-differentiated (Grade I, 50%), moderately differentiated (Grade II, 35%), and poorly differentiated (Grade III, 15%) tumors, depending on the dominant histologic pattern.[24] Most pathologists currently use the International Federation of Gynecology and Obstetrics grading system, which divides endometrial adenocarcinomas into three grades and correlates very well with the usual histologic classification. If the tumor is composed exclusively or almost exclusively of glands, with or without papillary elements, it is designated Grade I. If the tumor grows predominantly in a glandular pattern but with a significant admixture of the solid-growth pattern, it is designated Grade II. If more than 50% of the tumor grows as solid sheets of anaplastic cells, the designation is Grade III. Estrogen and progesterone receptors, as detected by biochemical analysis or immunocytochemistry, have also been studied in endometrial adenocarcinomas. The hormone receptor–positive tumors tend to be better-differentiated adenocarcinoma, often accompanied by endometrial hyperplasia, and are associated with a better prognosis.[6,9,12,20]

Well-Differentiated Adenocarcinoma

This type of tumor usually grows on the surface and only invades the uterine wall as a late event. Microscopically, there is an overabundance of glands, which are crowded against each other with only very thin bands of stroma separating them. A prominent infolding of the lining epithelium is usually noted. In some areas, the tumor is formed of cylindrical cells with elongated, hyperchromatic nuclei. Stratification of tumor cells is present in some of the glands. The nuclei are enlarged, with frequent small or prominent nucleoli. Mitoses may be numerous. Stromal cells are scant and retain their spindle shape, appearing fibroblast-like. Bundles of collagen fibers insinuate among them in all directions.

In endometrial brushing preparations obtained by direct endometrial sampling, abundant tumor cells occur singly, in loose groupings, or in three-dimensional, cohesive groupings with disorganized arrangements against a background of mucoid material. Tumor diathesis consisting of necrotic cellular debris, red blood cells, and inflammatory cells is usually present. The tumor cells often show variation in nuclear size. Their nuclei are round and ovoid, and many of them are enlarged. They have slightly coarse or coarsely granular chromatin and frequent conspicuous nucleoli (Images 5.1–5.4). Some of the tumor cells contain vacuolated cytoplasm, which are periodic acid-Schiff– and mucicarmine-positive, indicating mucin-producing activity. It is not uncommon that the mucin vacuoles within the cytoplasm contain neutrophils, which are readily visualized during the screening of the smears (Images 5.5–5.7). The amount of cytoplasm is variable among different tumor cells within the same tumor. The average amount of cytoplasm is also variable among different tumors. In some tumors, the neoplastic cells contain more abundant cytoplasm than those seen in other tumors (Images 5.8–5.12). The stromal cells are usually scant and appear fibroblast-like. Clusters of stromal foam cells may be observed (Images 5.13–5.16).

Moderately Differentiated Adenocarcinoma

Moderately differentiated adenocarcinoma presents glands with more irregular contours and solid cell nests or masses. The size of these glands and cell nests varies greatly. The glands often assume a papillary aspect, and the glandular epithelia show pronounced cellular atypia. Mitotic figures are numerous. The stroma appears desmoplastic. Stromal foam cells may be present.

In endometrial brushing preparations, the tumor cells lie singly, or occur in loose groups or cohesive groupings with disorganized arrangements. They have enlarged nuclei with frequent prominent nucleoli and a small to moderate amount of cytoplasm. The nuclei exhibit marked variations in size and shape, and have coarsely granular chromatin. Tumor cells with vacuolated cytoplasm containing neutrophils may also be present. Mitotic figures are easy to find (Images 5.17–5.22). Fibroblast-looking stromal cells are noticed. Clusters of stromal foam cells may be seen.

Poorly Differentiated Adenocarcinoma

This type of tumor invades the myometrium rapidly. Histologically, glandular formations have mostly disappeared. The tumor cells are disposed in nests or large sheets and manifest bizarre atypical forms. Their nuclei are irregular, hyperchromatic, and voluminous. Tumor necrosis is a common finding. Mitoses are abundant and atypical. The stroma is minimal in amount and is infiltrated by neutrophils and histiocytes.

In endometrial brushing preparations, large, pleomorphic tumor cells lie singly, or occur in loose groups or occasionally in cohesive, disorganized groupings. The background usually consists of necrotic debris intermixed with neutrophils, red blood cells, and histiocytes. The tumor cells are large and some have high nuclear/cytoplasmic ratios. Their nuclei are also enlarged and appear irregular, with coarsely granular chromatin and frequent prominent nucleoli (Images 5.23–5.27). Atypical mitotic figures are present. The stromal cells have fusiform nuclei and scant, ill-defined cytoplasm, and are relatively rare. Stromal foam cells may be present.

Cytologic Differentiation Between Severe Hyperplasia and Well-Differentiated Adenocarcinoma

The cytologic diagnosis of moderately differentiated or poorly differentiated endometrial adenocarcinoma based on endometrial brushing preparations is usually straightforward. However, the cytologic diagnosis of well-differentiated adenocarcinoma of the endometrium as opposed to severe endometrial hyperplasia is not always straightforward. In the interpretation of endometrial brushing preparations, the key features that should be carefully investigated include:

1. Cellularity and number of cell clusters. This is particularly important in postmenopausal women whose endometrial brushing preparations are usually scantily cellular. An endometrial brushing preparation from a postmenopausal woman containing abundant cells or cell clusters may indicate a significant abnormality.
2. Cellular arrangements. Benign glandular cells are usually in sheet arrangements in brushing preparations. The presence of many three-dimensional, disorganized cell groupings and overcrowding flat sheets of atypical glandular cells is highly suggestive of malignancy, and unlikely for endometrial hyperplasia.
3. Cohesion between glandular cells. Benign glandular cells have good intercellular cohesions and occur in sheet arrangements in brushing preparations. Breakdown of cell clusters into solitary cells and small loose groupings is common in malignant tumors and unusual in endometrial hyperplasia.
4. Background material. Mucoid background is observed in endometrial samples procured during the secretory phase and also in cases of endometrial adenocarcinoma in brushing preparations (best seen in direct smear preparations), and is rarely seen in samples from postmenopausal women with endometrial hyperplasia. However, tumor diathesis consisting of necrotic cellular debris, red blood cells, and inflammatory cells intermixed with mucoid material is only seen in malignant conditions.
5. Stromal foam cells. These cells are rarely observed in benign conditions of the endometrium, and therefore, their presence serves to warn of endometrial hyperplasia or endometrial carcinoma. They often occur in cohesive clusters; this cytologic feature distinguishes them from foamy histiocytes, which virtually always lie singly in brushing preparations. However, the stromal foam cells seen in endometrial hyperplasias are morphologically identical to those present in endometrial adenocarcinomas.
6. Atypical glandular cells. The highly atypical glandular cells have very large nuclei with coarse chromatin and prominent nucleoli, and show nuclear pleomorphism, almost always indicating adenocarcinoma. However, these cells are only seen in poorly differentiated tumors. The finding of many disorganized groupings of glandular cells showing conspicuous nucleoli and some variation in nuclear size is also

No single pathognomonic feature distinguishes well-differentiated adenocarcinoma from severe hyperplasia

Table 5.1
Cytologic Differentiation Between Severe Endometrial Hyperplasia
and Well-Differentiated Adenocarcinoma

Cytologic Findings	Severe Hyperplasia	Well-Differentiated Adenocarcinoma
Cellular arrangements	Sheets, cohesive groupings (flat)	Solitary cells, loose groups, 3-D cohesive groupings (disordered)
Cytoplasm		
Abundance	Usually scant	A small amount to abundant
Vacuolation	Nonvacuolated	Some tumor cells with vacuolated cytoplasm often containing neutrophils
Nuclei		
Size	Small to medium	Small to large
Nucleoli	Inconspicuous, rarely prominent	Inconspicuous, often prominent
Chromatin	Slightly coarse	Slightly coarse or coarsely granular
Tumor diathesis	Absent	Usually present
Mucoid background	Rare	Often seen
Stromal cells	Spindle cells with plump nuclei	Fibroblast-looking

consistent with malignancy. Overemphasizing the significance of nuclear enlargement is misleading. The average nuclear size of glandular cells in some cases of endometrial hyperplasia is larger than that in many cases of well-differentiated adenocarcinoma. Overemphasizing the significance of conspicuous nucleoli is also misleading. Conspicuous nucleoli may be seen in glandular cells during the late proliferative or secretory phase, and are also seen in cases of endometrial hyperplasia. Prominent nucleoli are often seen in predecidual cells.

7. Mucin-secreting activity. The finding of clusters of mucin-secreting cells with multivacuolated cytoplasm often infiltrated with neutrophils is highly suggestive of adenocarcinoma, and not consistent with endometrial hyperplasia. The secretory glandular cells during the secretory phase show only clear cytoplasm in endometrial brushing preparations, and do not appear multivacuolated.

The cytologic diagnosis of an endometrial carcinoma should be based on overall findings. The cytologic differentiation between severe endometrial hyperplasia and well-differentiated adenocarcinoma is sometimes difficult, especially when the specimen is scant; however, in a good brushing preparation with cellular material there are cytologic features that can be used to differentiate these two conditions (Table 5.1).

Adenocarcinoma With Squamous Differentiation

Endometrial adenocarcinomas containing squamous elements are common, but the amount of squamous epithelium varies widely. Adenocarcinoma with squamous elements can be divided into those with benign-appearing squamous differentiation (adenoacanthoma or adeno-carcinoma with squamous metaplasia) and those with malignant squamous epithelium (adenosquamous carcinoma).[18] Women with adenoacanthoma are more often premenopausal and slightly younger than women with adenosquamous carcinoma (mean age of 58 years). These neoplasms differ markedly in their behavior; the 5-year survival for adenosquamous carcinoma is 19% to 40% compared with about 70% to 80% for adenoacanthoma. Thus, adenoacanthoma is a relatively well-differentiated carcinoma with an excellent prognosis, whereas adenosquamous carcinoma is poorly differentiated carcinoma with an unfavorable outlook.[1,25,28] Pure squamous carcinoma of the endometrium is extremely rare.

Adenoacanthoma

Adenoacanthoma (adenocarcinoma with squamous metaplasia) is characterized by a mixture of adenocarcinoma and squamous epithelium arising in the glands. The squamous epithelium is cytologically benign and the malignant glandular component is usually well-differentiated. The nests of squamous epithelium are usually confined to gland lumina. The squamous epithelium resembles metaplastic squamous cells of the cervical transformation zone.

In endometrial brushing preparations, two populations of tumor cells are noted. Groups of tumor cells resembling those from well-differentiated endometrial adenocarcinoma intermix with or in direct continuity with groups of large tumor cells with an abundance of dense cytoplasm, resembling metaplastic squamous cells. Adenocarcinoma cells usually predominate (Images 5.28–5.31). Other cytologic findings are more or less the same as those in cases of endometrial adenocarcinoma of the well-differentiated type.

Adenosquamous Carcinoma

Adenosquamous carcinoma is defined as an adenocarcinoma that also contains malignant squamous epithelium. The squamous element is cytologically malignant and is not confined to gland lumina but often extends out from the glands. It may not be in direct continuity with the glandular epithelium, appearing in isolated nests. Keratinization and epithelial pearl formation occur to varying degrees. Both of the glandular and squamous components display nuclear atypia and increased mitotic activity. The malignant glandular component is usually moderately or poorly differentiated, and the neoplastic glandular cells show an increased nuclear/cytoplasmic ratio.

In endometrial brushing preparations, malignant glandular cells of the moderately or poorly differentiated type intermix with malignant squamous cells, which are usually of the nonkeratinizing type that have large, pleomorphic nuclei with coarsely granular chromatin and abundant dense cytoplasm (Images 5.32–5.35). Malignant squamous cells of the keratinizing type are less frequently encountered. These cells usually have pyknotic nuclei and an abundance of well-defined, dense, orangeo-philic cytoplasm. Epithelial pearls in whorl arrangements may be seen (Images 5.36–5.39).

Clear Cell Carcinoma

Clear cell carcinoma is a distinctive type of endometrial carcinoma similar to those that occur in the ovary, vagina, and cervix. It occurs in older women (mean age, 67 years) and has an unfavorable prognosis. Histologically, clear cell carcinoma may exhibit solid, papillary, tubular, and cystic patterns. The clear cytoplasm is due largely to the presence of glycogen.[4,11] Cystic spaces are frequently lined by flattened cells. Psammoma bodies can be found in association with papillary areas within the tumor.

In endometrial brushing preparations, the tumor cells occur in cohesive groupings or as solitary cells. They are typically large, with clear or lightly stained cytoplasm by Papanicolaou stain. Nuclear atypia is generally marked, manifested by pleomorphism and large nuclei with prominent nucleoli (Images 5.40–5.42). Mitotic activity is high and abnormal mitotic figures are often seen. Intracellular and extracellular hyaline bodies, which are periodic acid-Schiff–positive and diastase-resistant, are often encountered.

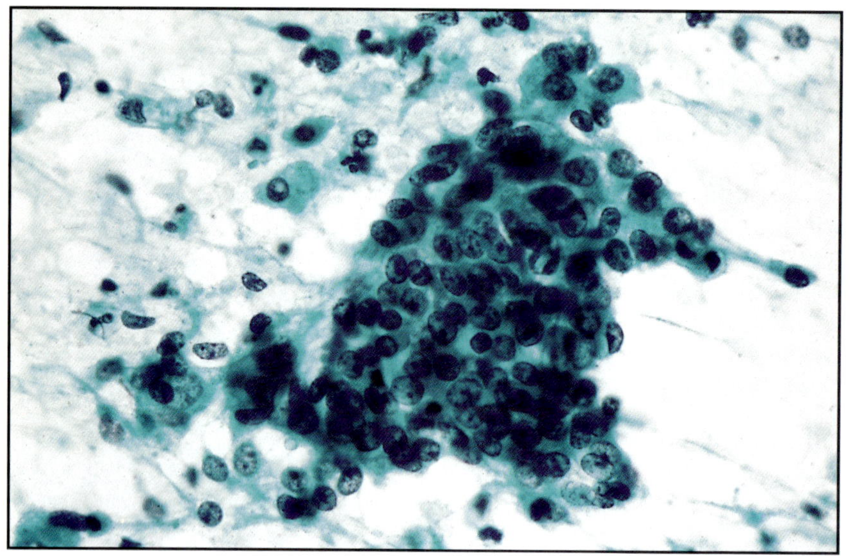

Image 5.1
Well-differentiated adenocarcinoma of the endometrium. The malignant cells have enlarged nuclei with prominent nucleoli and slightly coarse chromatin and various amounts of cytoplasm. They occur in a three-dimensional grouping. Variation in nuclear size is evident. Endometrial brushing (Papanicolaou, 400X).

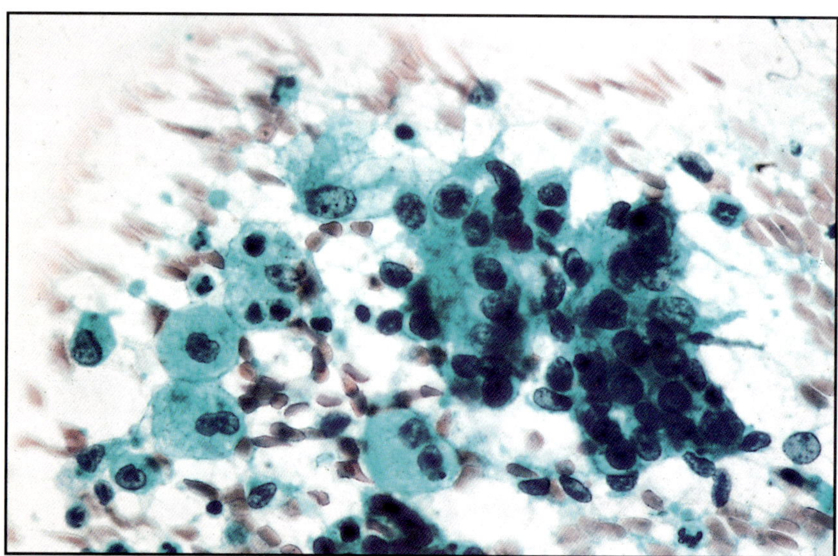

Image 5.2
Well-differentiated adenocarcinoma of the endometrium. The malignant cells have hyperchromatic nuclei and scant, ill-defined cytoplasm, and occur as solitary cells or in loose groupings. Endometrial brushing (Papanicolaou, 400X).

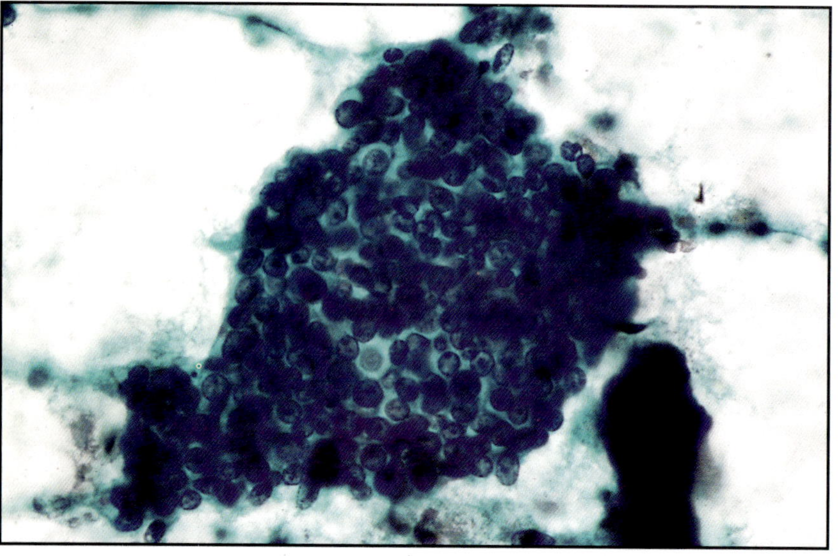

Image 5.3
Well-differentiated adenocarcinoma of the endometrium. The malignant cells have hyperchromatic nuclei with frequent prominent nucleoli and marked variation in nuclear size, and occur in a three-dimensional grouping with disordered arrangements. Endometrial brushing (Papanicolaou, 400X).

Image 5.4
Well-differentiated adenocarcinoma of the endometrium. The malignant cells have hyperchromatic nuclei with frequent prominent nucleoli and coarse chromatin, and occur in tightly packed, three-dimensional groupings. Endometrial brushing (Papanicolaou, 400X).

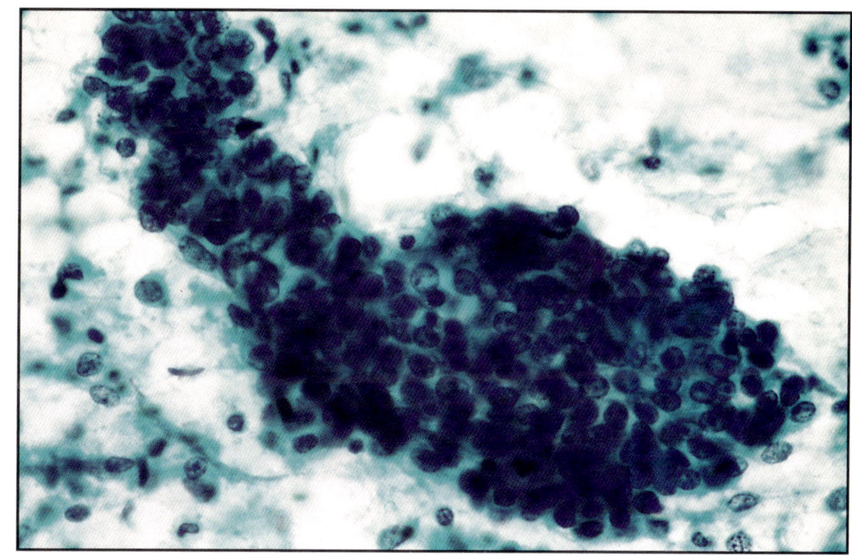

Image 5.5
Well-differentiated adenocarcinoma of the endometrium. The malignant cells have an abundance of vacuolated cytoplasm, indicating mucin-secreting activity. Note that the background appears mucoid. Endometrial brushing (Papanicolaou, 400X).

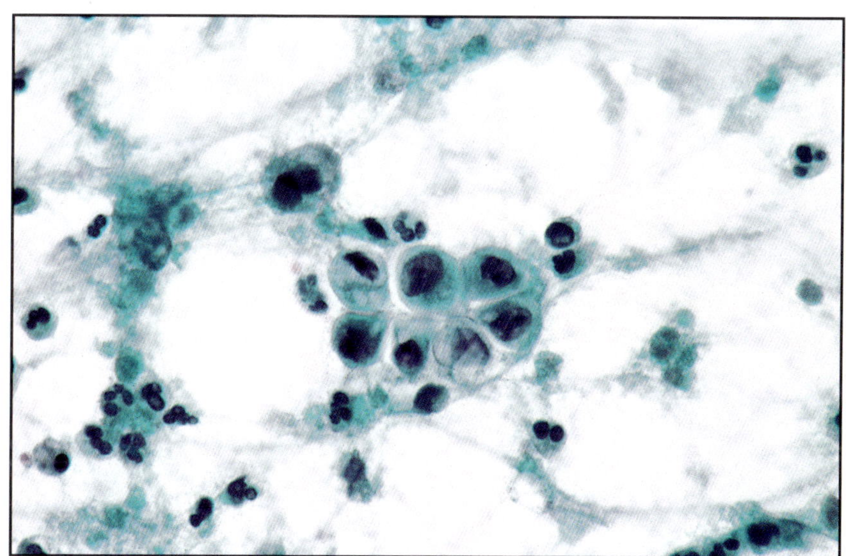

Image 5.6
Well-differentiated adenocarcinoma of the endometrium. Some of the mucin vacuoles within the cytoplasm of the malignant cells contain neutrophils. This is a common finding in mucin-secreting adenocarcinoma and is readily visualized during the screening of brushing smears. Endometrial brushing (Papanicolaou, 400X).

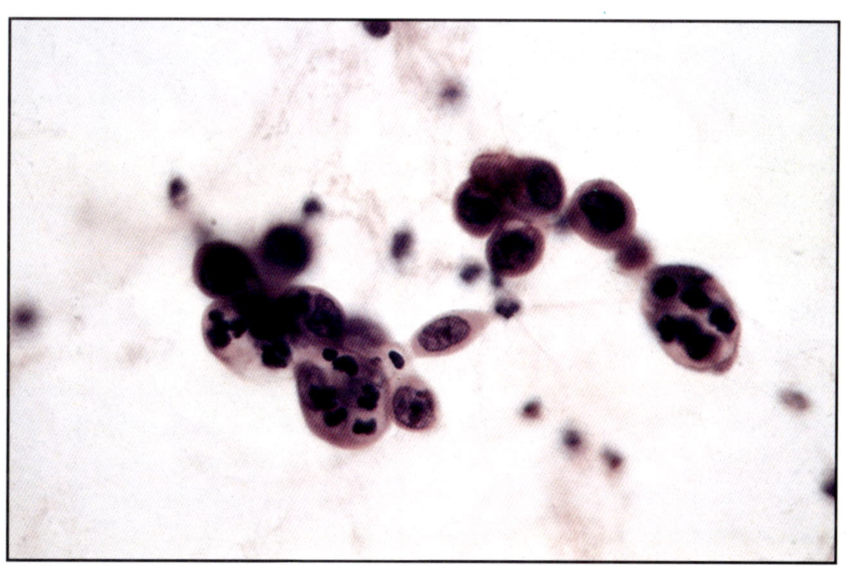

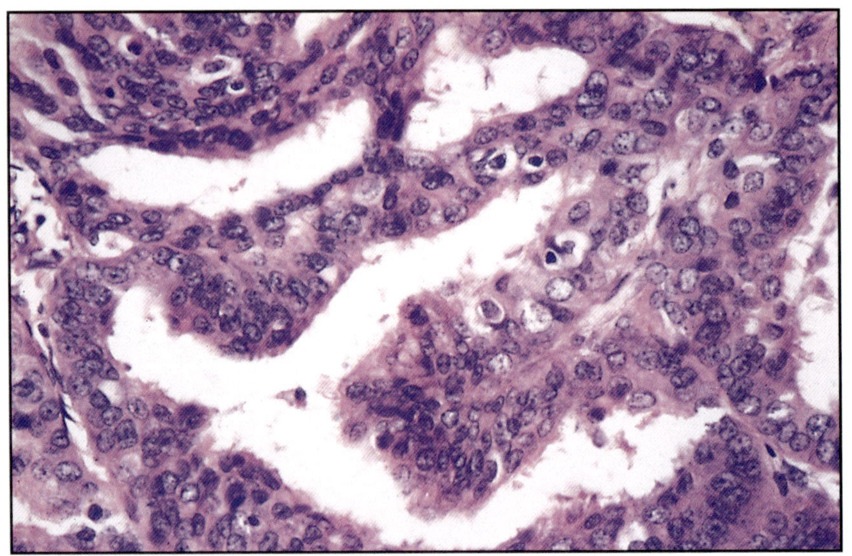

Image 5.7
Well-differentiated adenocarcinoma of the endometrium. The tumor is composed of glandular cells with hyperchromatic nuclei and frequent prominent nucleoli. The glands are crowded against each other. A prominent infolding of the lining epithelium is noted. The nuclei are enlarged, and stratification of tumor cells is present. Histologic section (H&E, 200X).

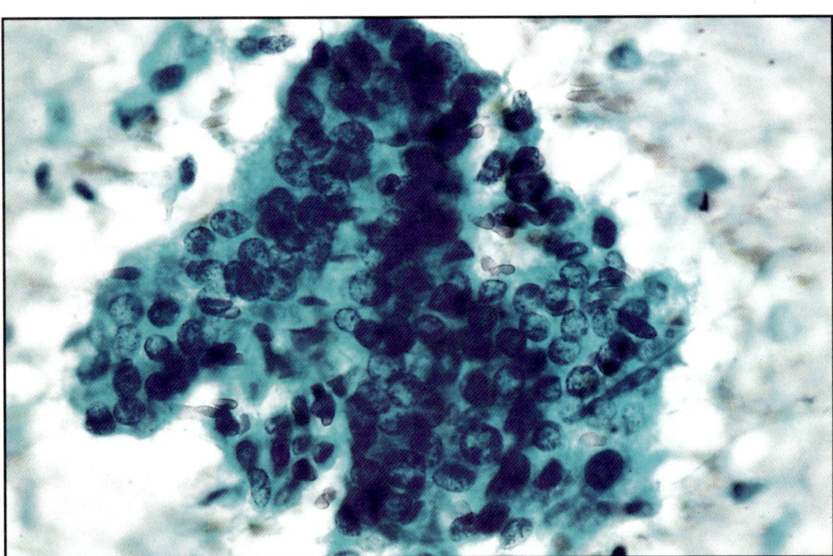

Image 5.8
Well-differentiated adenocarcinoma of the endometrium. The malignant cells have enlarged nuclei and a moderate amount to an abundance of cytoplasm. They occur in three-dimensional, disordered groupings. Endometrial brushing (Papanicolaou, 400X).

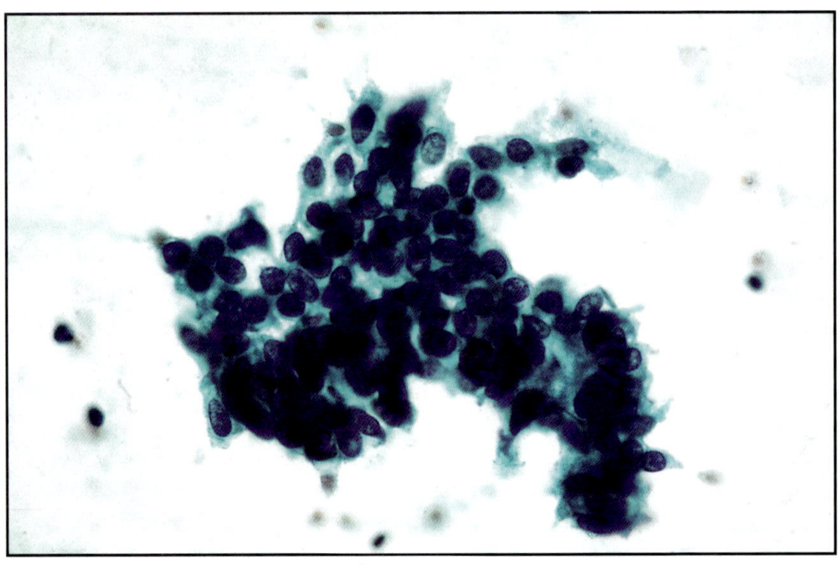

Image 5.9
Well-differentiated adenocarcinoma of the endometrium. The malignant cells have hyperchromatic nuclei and a moderate amount of cytoplasm, and occur in loosely packed groupings. Endometrial brushing (Papanicolaou, 400X).

Image 5.10
Well-differentiated adenocarcinoma of
the endometrium. The malignant cells
have hyperchromatic nuclei and various
amount of cytoplasm, and occur in
tightly packed, three-dimensional groupings. Endometrial brushing (Papanicolaou, 400X).

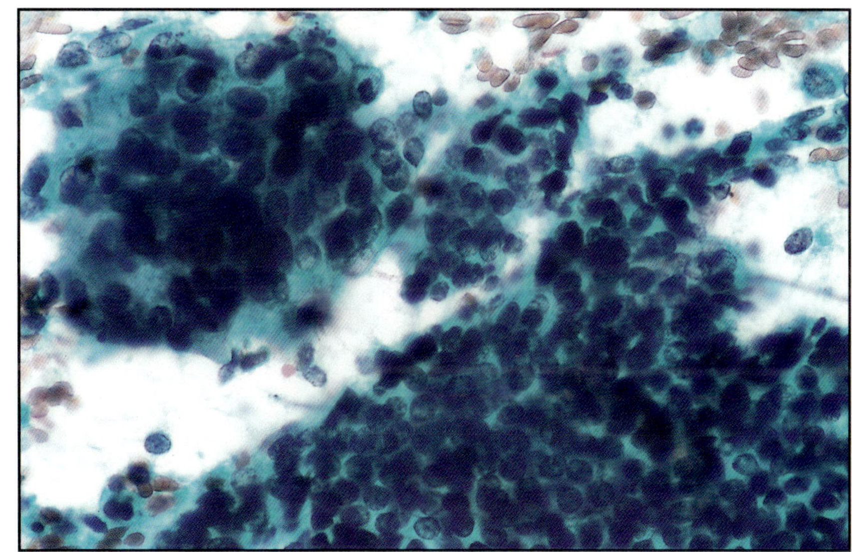

Image 5.11
Well-differentiated adenocarcinoma of
the endometrium. Two clusters of
closely packed malignant cells with
clear or vacuolated cytoplasm containing
neutrophils. Endometrial brushing
(Papanicolaou, 400X).

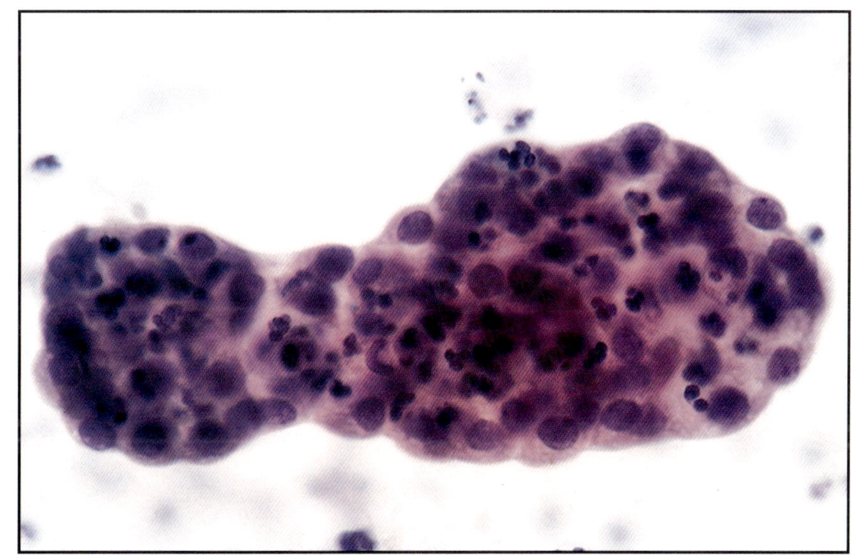

Image 5.12
Well-differentiated adenocarcinoma of
the endometrium. There is an overabundance of glands, which are crowded
against each other with only thin bands
of stroma separating them. The tumor
is composed of glandular cells containing
more abundant cytoplasm (as compared
with the tumor cells shown in Image
5.7), which correspond to the tumor
cells shown in Images 5.8 to 5.11. Histologic section (H&E, 200X).

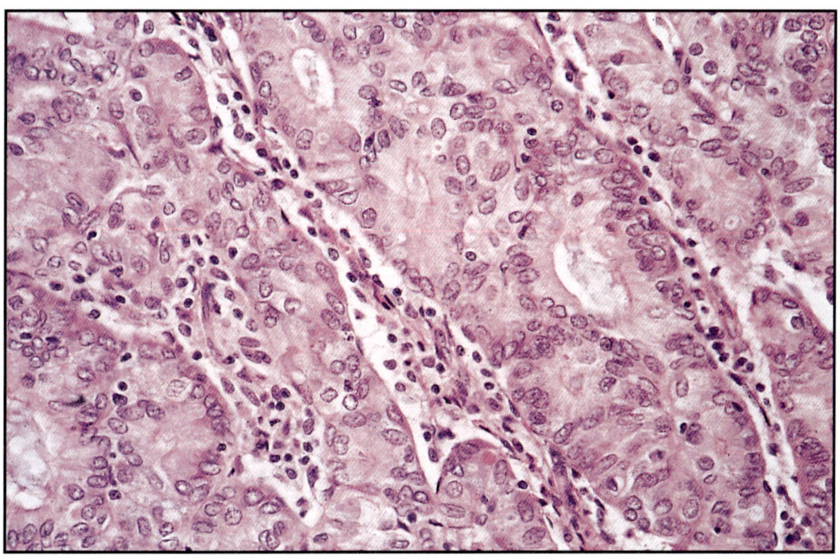

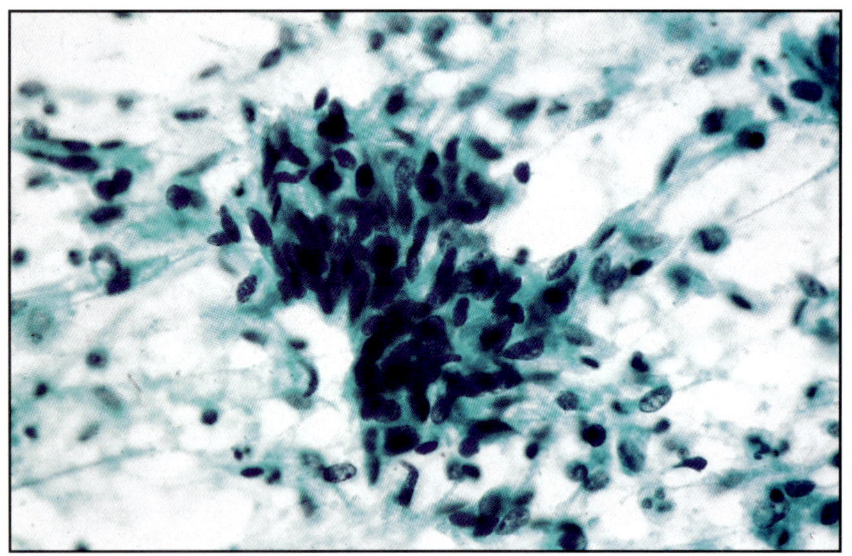

Image 5.13
Stromal cells in adenocarcinoma of the endometrium. The stromal cells have fusiform nuclei and relatively scant, ill-defined cytoplasm, and occur in cohesive groupings. Their appearance is fibroblast-like. Endometrial brushing (Papanicolaou, 400X).

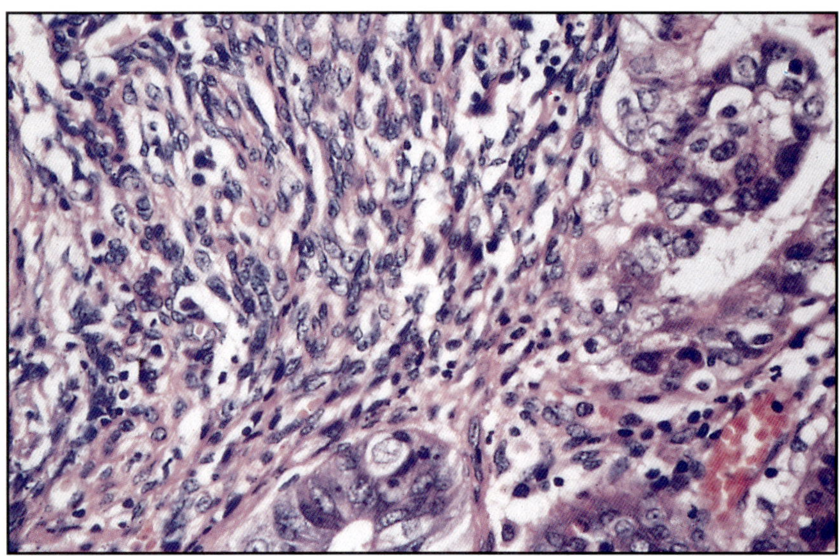

Image 5.14
Stromal cells in adenocarcinoma of the endometrium. The stromal cells retain their spindle shape, appearing fibroblast-like (see Image 5.13). They are relatively scant in the tumor. Histologic section (H&E, 200X).

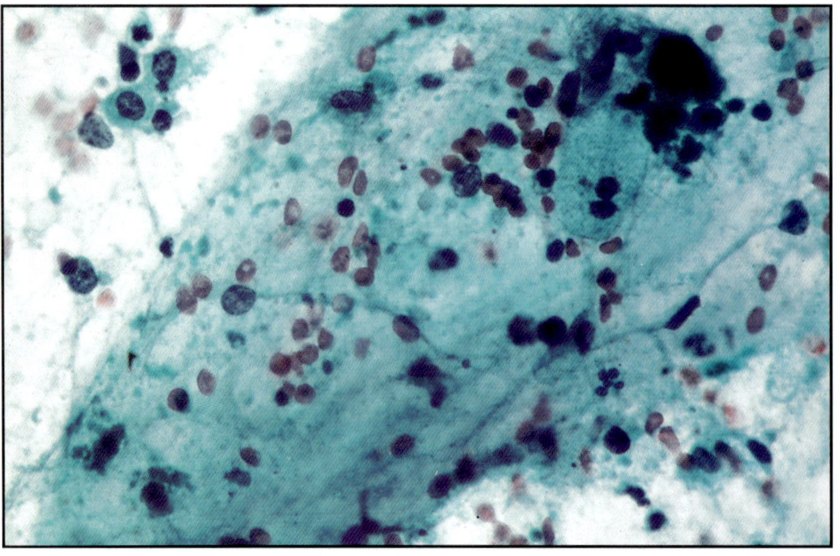

Image 5.15
Tumor diathesis in adenocarcinoma of the endometrium. Abundant mucoid material admixes with necrotic cellular debris, red blood cells, and inflammatory cells. Endometrial brushing (Papanicolaou, 400X).

Image 5.16
Stromal foam cells in adenocarcinoma of the endometrium. The stromal foam cells have large ovoid, vesicular nuclei and an abundance of foamy cytoplasm. They occur in a cohesive grouping. Endometrial brushing (Papanicolaou, 400X).

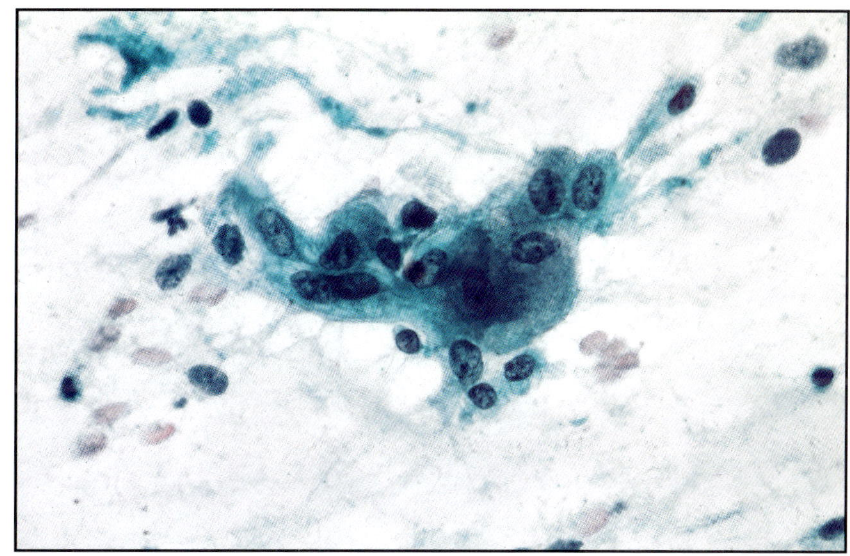

Image 5.17
Moderately differentiated adenocarcinoma of the endometrium. The malignant cells have pleomorphic, hyperchromatic nuclei with coarsely granular chromatin and a small amount of cytoplasm, and occur in loose groupings. Endometrial brushing (Papanicolaou, 400X).

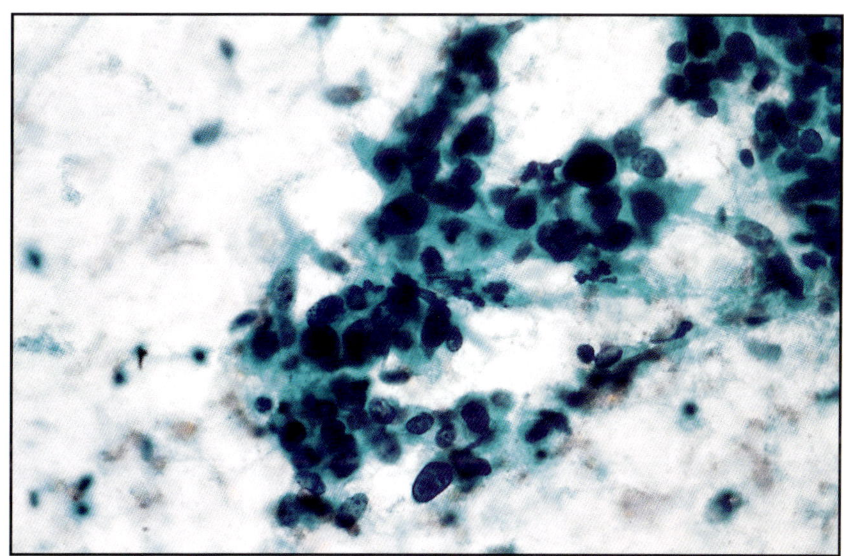

Image 5.18
Moderately differentiated adenocarcinoma of the endometrium. The malignant cells have relatively large nuclei with coarse chromatin and prominent nucleoli and a small to moderate amount of cytoplasm. They occur in disordered groupings. Endometrial brushing (Papanicolaou, 400X).

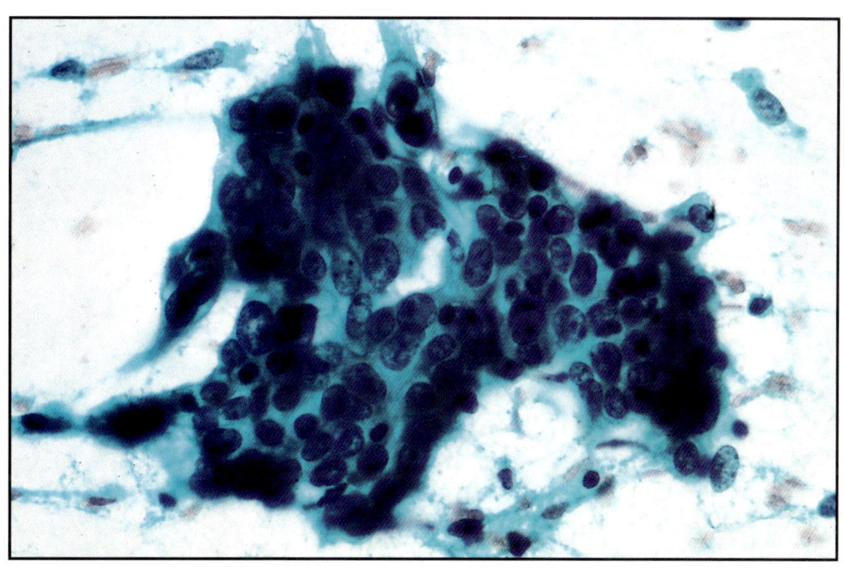

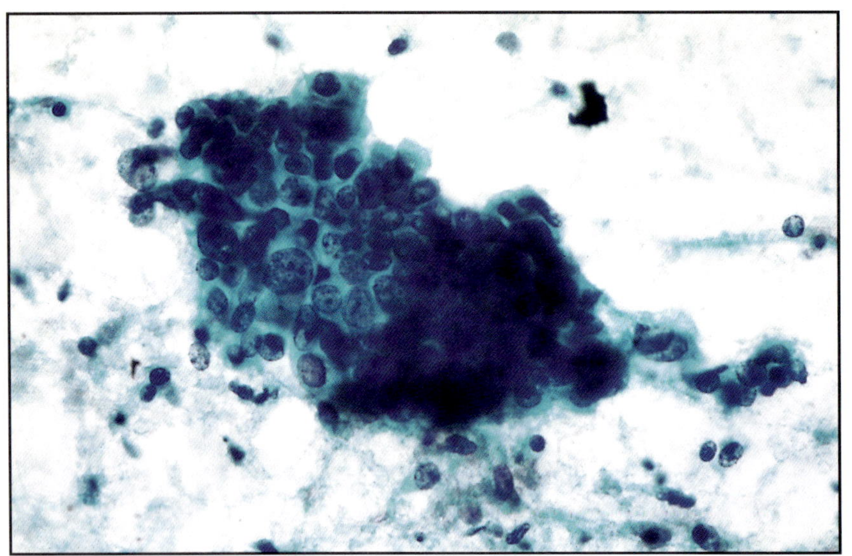

Image 5.19
Moderately differentiated adenocarcinoma of the endometrium. The malignant cells have pleomorphic nuclei and relatively scant cytoplasm, and occur in a tightly packed, three-dimensional, disorganized grouping. Endometrial brushing (Papanicolaou, 400X).

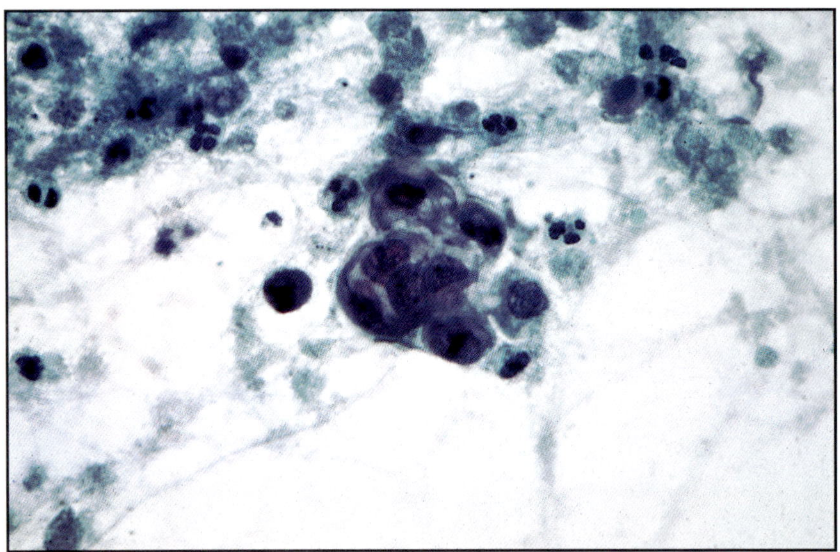

Image 5.20
Moderately differentiated adenocarcinoma of the endometrium. A loose group of malignant cells that have an abundance of vacuolated cytoplasm and large nuclei with coarsely granular chromatin is present against a mucoid background. Endometrial brushing (Papanicolaou, 400X).

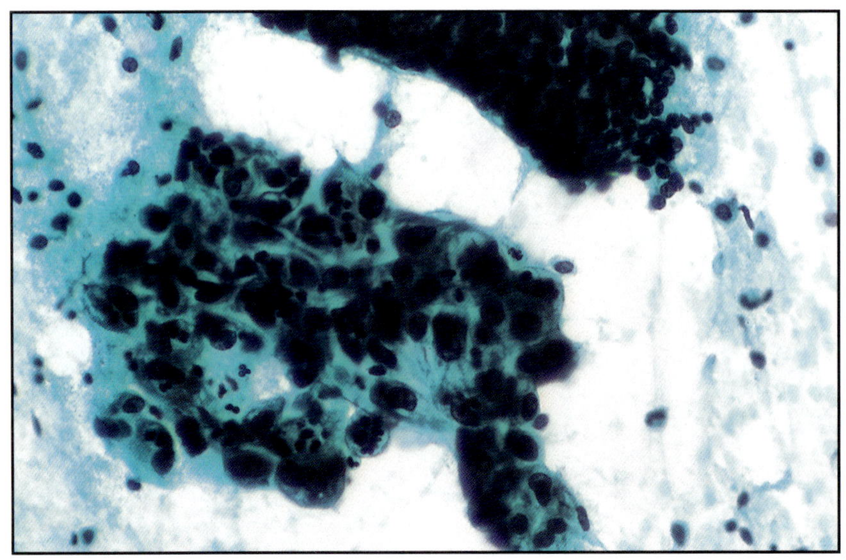

Image 5.21
Moderately differentiated adenocarcinoma of the endometrium. A cohesive grouping of malignant cells that have hyperchromatic nuclei and a moderate amount of cytoplasm is infiltrated by neutrophils. Endometrial brushing (Papanicolaou, 400X).

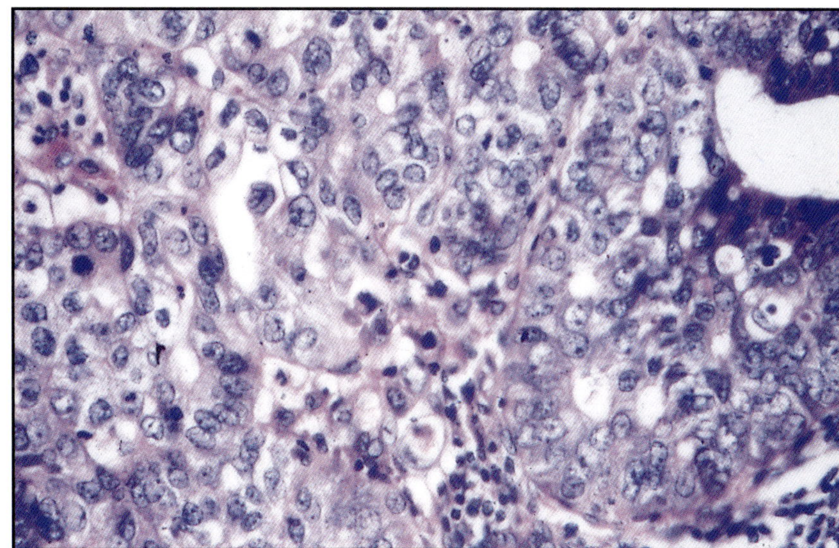

Image 5.22
Moderately differentiated adenocarcinoma of the endometrium. The tumor consists of glands with irregular contours and solid nests or masses of neoplastic cells. The glandular epithelia show pronounced cellular atypia. Mitotic figures are numerous. Histologic section (H&E, 200X).

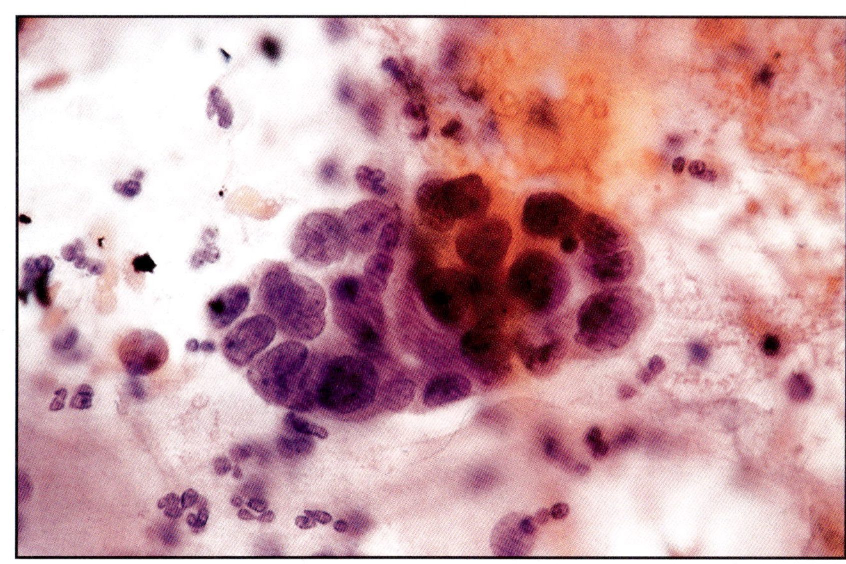

Image 5.23
Poorly differentiated adenocarcinoma of the endometrium. The malignant cells have large, irregular-shaped nuclei with coarse chromatin and scant cytoplasm, and occur in loose groupings. Endometrial brushing (Papanicolaou, 400X).

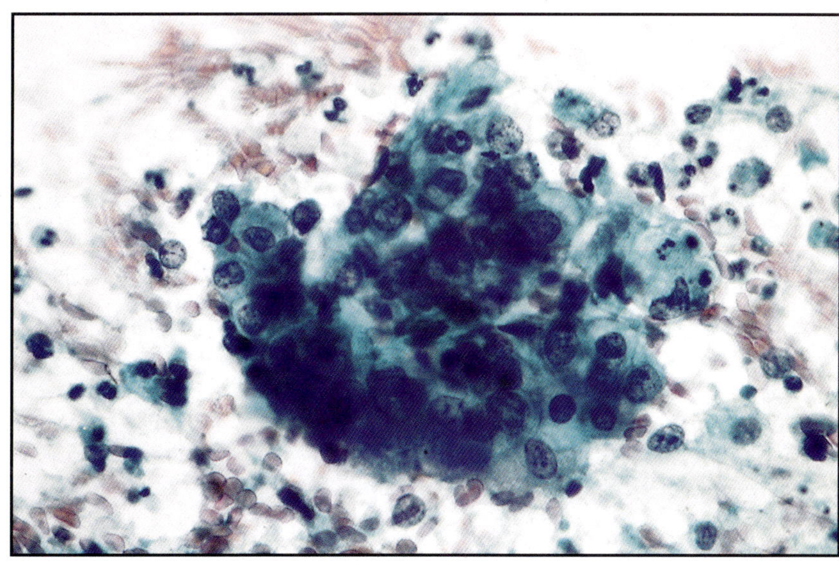

Image 5.24
Poorly differentiated adenocarcinoma of the endometrium. The malignant cells have pleomorphic nuclei with coarse chromatin and various amounts of cytoplasm, and occur in disorganized groupings. Endometrial brushing (Papanicolaou, 400X).

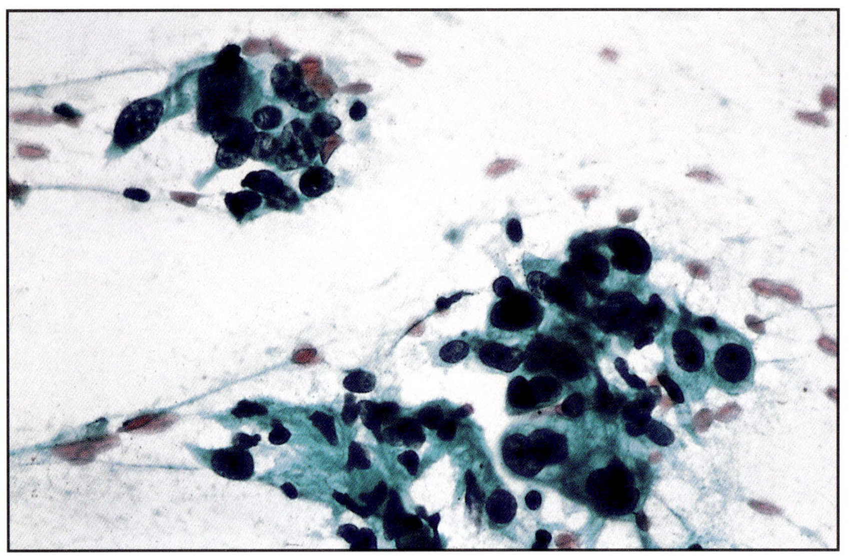

Image 5.25
Poorly differentiated adenocarcinoma of the endometrium. The malignant cells have large, pleomorphic, hyperchromatic nuclei with coarsely granular chromatin and various amounts of cytoplasm, and occur in loose groupings or as solitary cells. Endometrial brushing (Papanicolaou, 400X).

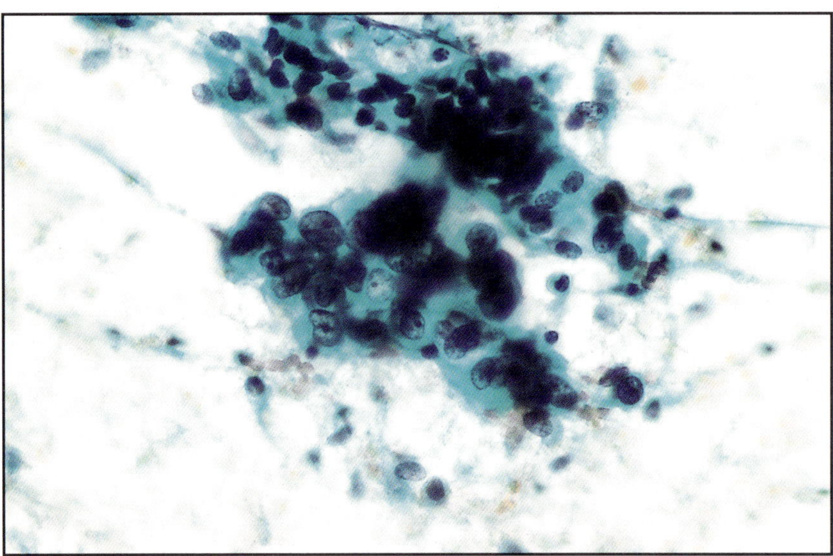

Image 5.26
Poorly differentiated adenocarcinoma of the endometrium. A loose group of malignant cells that have pleomorphic nuclei with prominent nucleoli intermingles with necrotic tumor debris. Endometrial brushing (Papanicolaou, 400X).

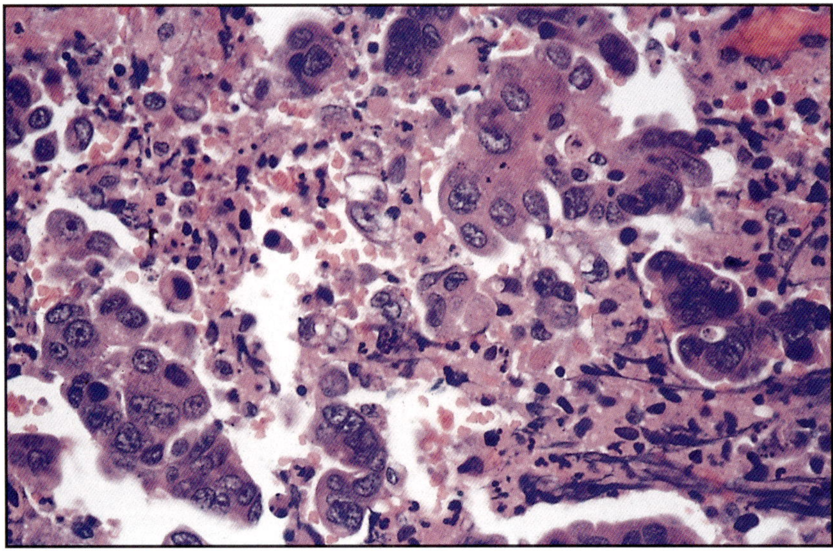

Image 5.27
Poorly differentiated adenocarcinoma of the endometrium. The tumor cells are disposed in nests or sheets and manifest bizarre atypical forms. Their nuclei are irregular, hyperchromatic, and voluminous. Glandular formations have disappeared. Histologic section (H&E, 200X).

Image 5.28
Adenoacanthoma of the endometrium.
A tightly packed, three-dimensional
grouping of malignant cells that have
enlarged nuclei with coarse chromatin
and scant cytoplasm resembles well-differentiated endometrial adenocarcinoma
(see Image 5.30). Endometrial brushing
(Papanicolaou, 400X).

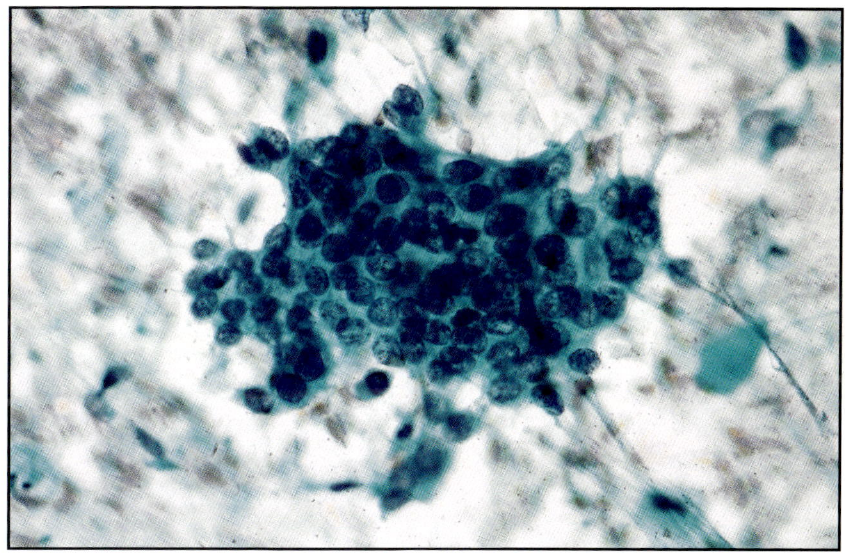

Image 5.29
Adenoacanthoma of the endometrium.
A disorganized grouping of malignant
cells that have nuclei with coarse chromatin and variable nuclear size and a
small amount of cytoplasm resembles
well-differentiated endometrial adenocarcinoma (see Image 5.30). Endometrial
brushing (Papanicolaou, 400X).

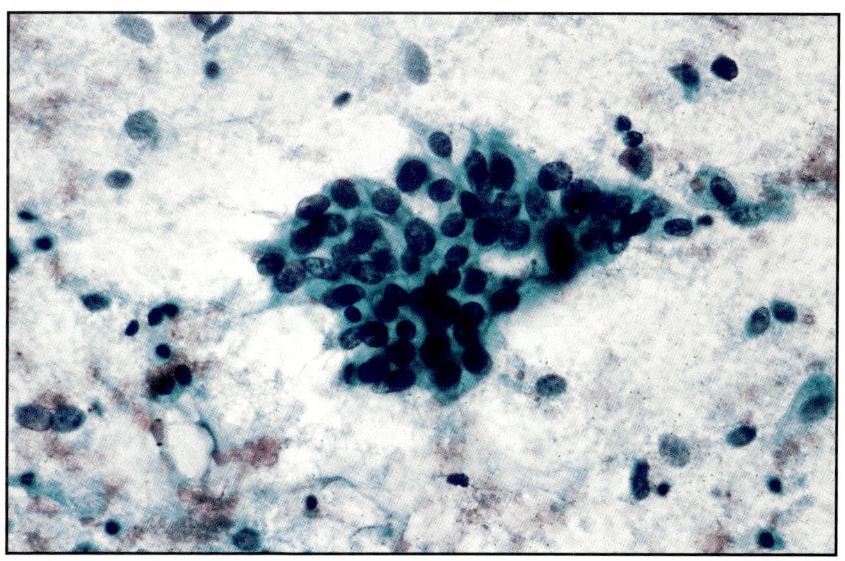

Image 5.30
Adenoacanthoma of the endometrium.
A few large cells that have an abundance of dense cytoplasm and centrally
located nuclei with fine chromatin
resemble metaplastic squamous cells of
the cervical transformation zone. Note
that these cells intermingle with adenocarcinoma cells seen in Images 5.28 and
5.29. Endometrial brushing (Papanicolaou, 400X).

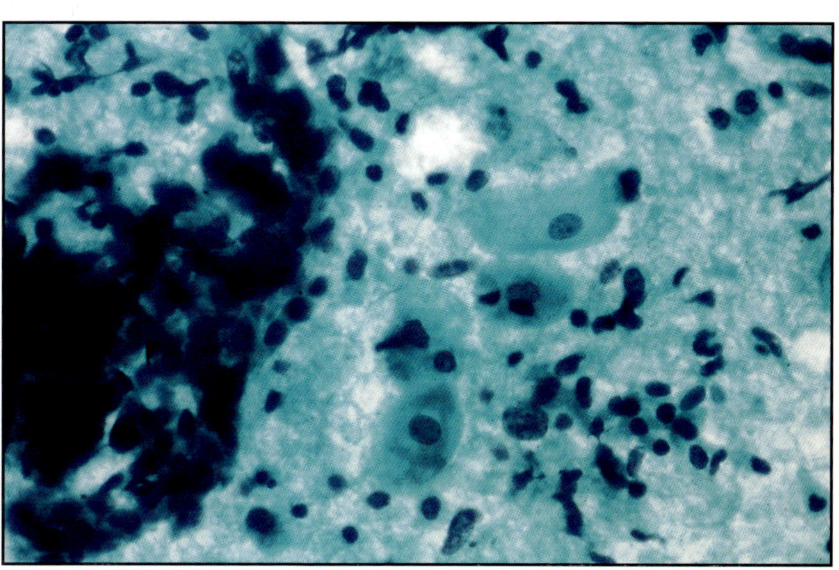

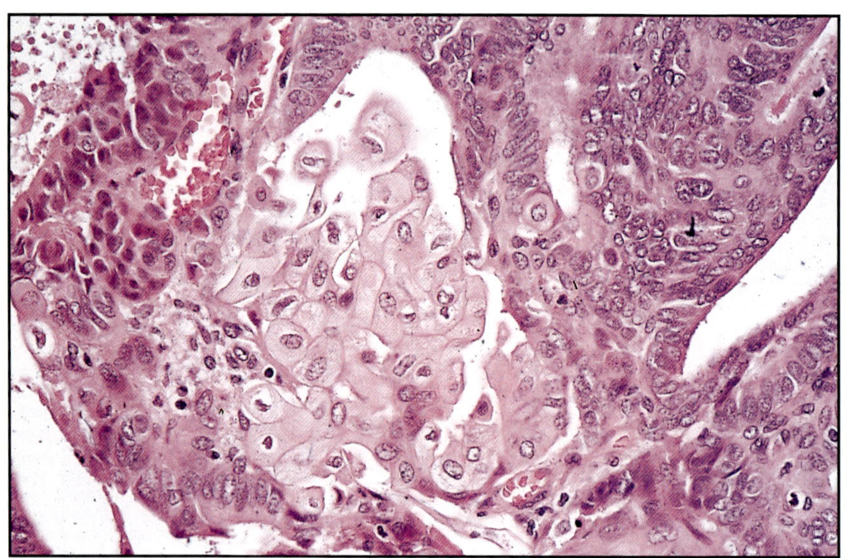

Image 5.31

Adenoacanthoma of the endometrium. The tumor is characterized by a mixture of adenocarcinoma and squamous epithelium arising in the glands. The squamous epithelium is cytologically benign, and the malignant glandular component is well-differentiated. Histologic section (H&E, 200X).

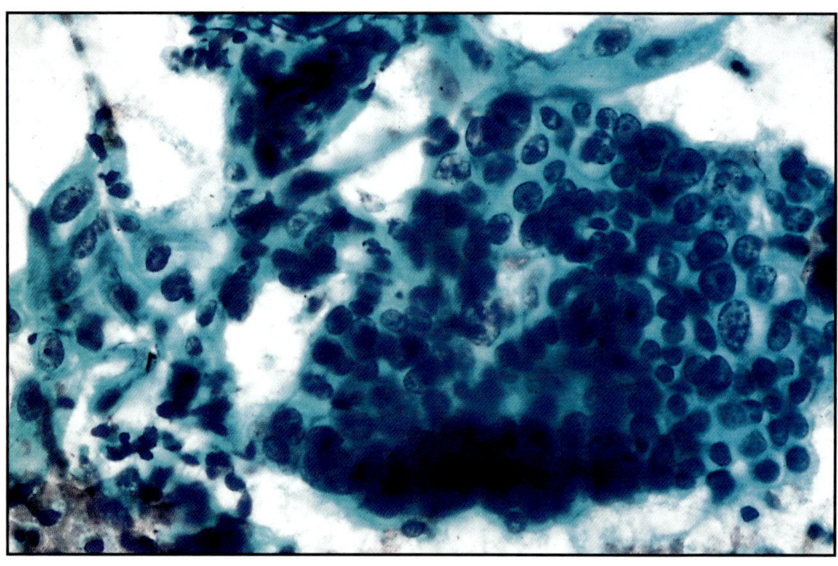

Image 5.32

Adenosquamous carcinoma of the endometrium. A disorganized grouping of malignant cells that have large, pleomorphic nuclei with coarse chromatin and prominent nucleoli and a small amount of cytoplasm resembles moderately differentiated endometrial adenocarcinoma (see Image 5.34). Endometrial brushing (Papanicolaou, 400X).

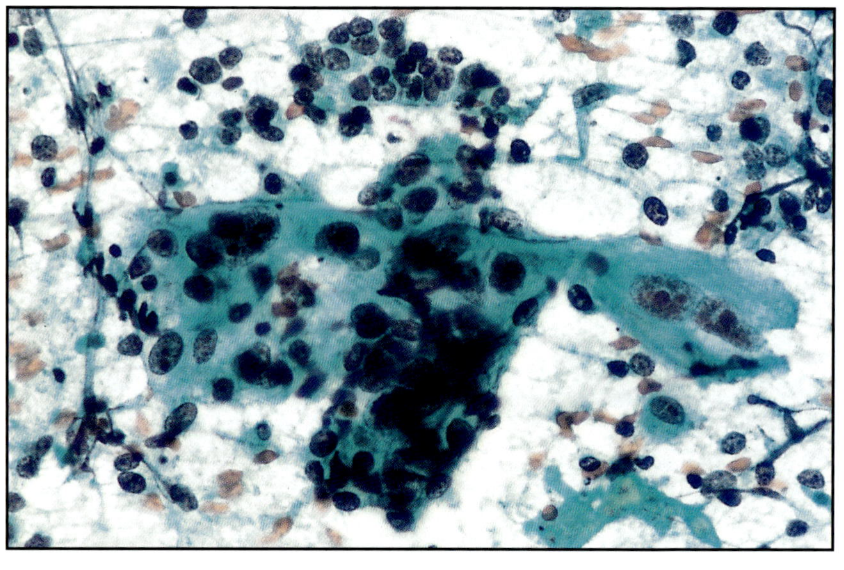

Image 5.33

Adenosquamous carcinoma of the endometrium. A few solitary adenocarcinoma cells intermingle with large malignant cells that have large, pleomorphic nuclei with coarsely granular chromatin and prominent nucleoli and an abundance of dense cytoplasm, resembling squamous cell carcinoma. Endometrial brushing (Papanicolaou, 400X).

Image 5.34
Adenosquamous carcinoma of the endometrium. Groups of malignant cells resembling those from adenocarcinoma of the endometrium are in direct continuity with groups of large malignant cells with an abundance of dense cytoplasm, resembling squamous cell carcinoma. Endometrial brushing (Papanicolaou, 400X).

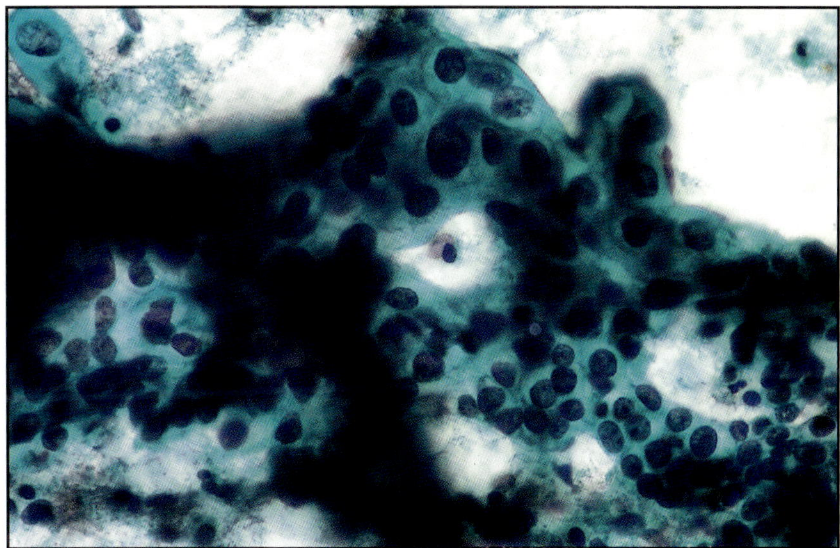

Image 5.35
Adenosquamous carcinoma of the endometrium. The tumor is characterized by a mixture of adenocarcinoma and squamous cell carcinoma. The malignant squamous component is of the nonkeratinizing type, and the malignant glandular component is moderately differentiated. Histologic section (H&E, 200X).

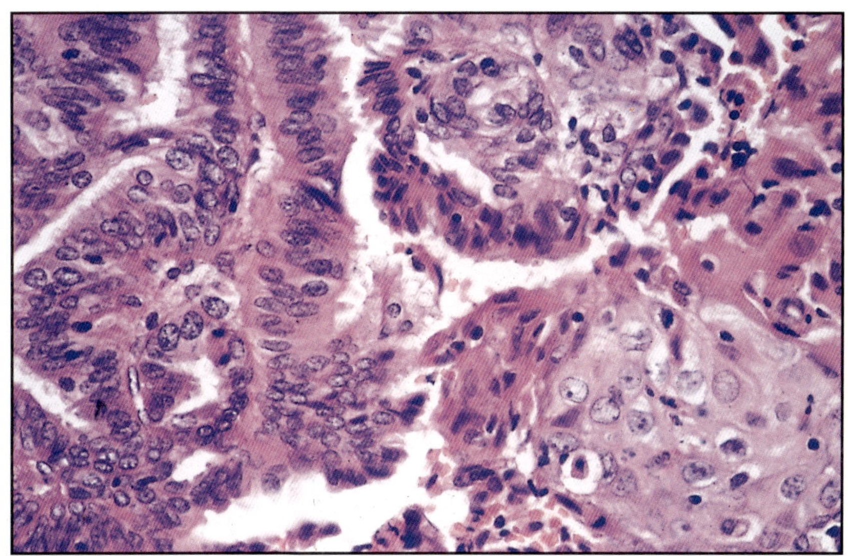

Image 5.36
Adenosquamous carcinoma of the endometrium. A loose group of malignant cells that have large, pleomorphic nuclei with coarse chromatin and scant cytoplasm resembles poorly differentiated endometrial adenocarcinoma (see Images 5.37 and 5.38). Endometrial brushing (Papanicolaou, 400X).

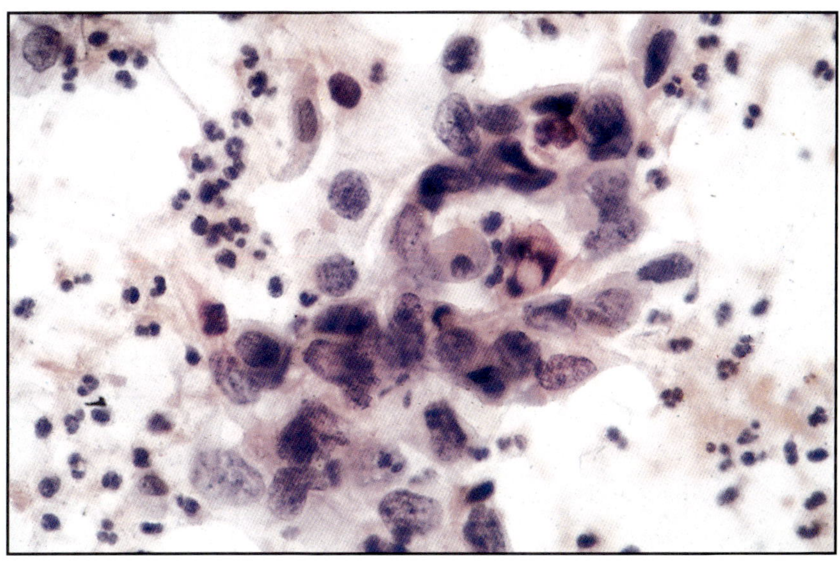

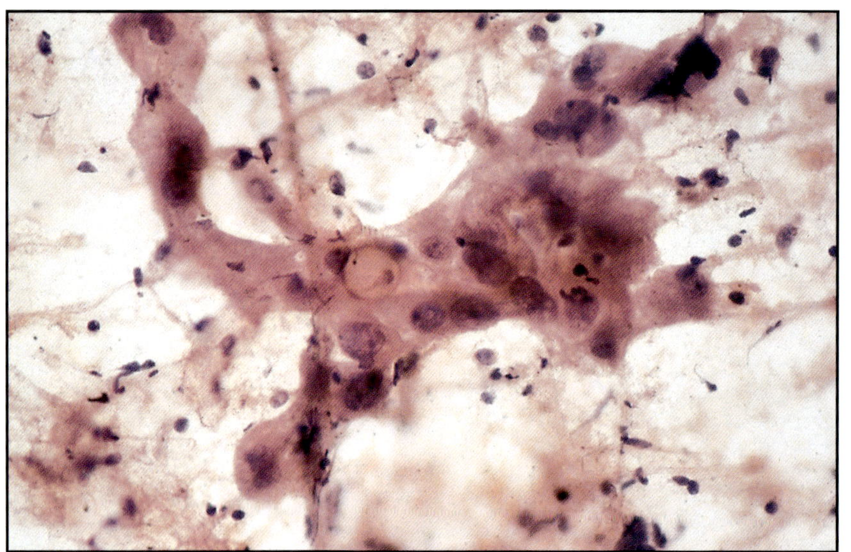

Image 5.37
Adenosquamous carcinoma of the endometrium. A cohesive grouping of large malignant cells that have an abundance of dense, eosinophilic cytoplasm resembles keratinizing squamous cell carcinoma (see Image 5.36). Endometrial brushing (Papanicolaou, 400X).

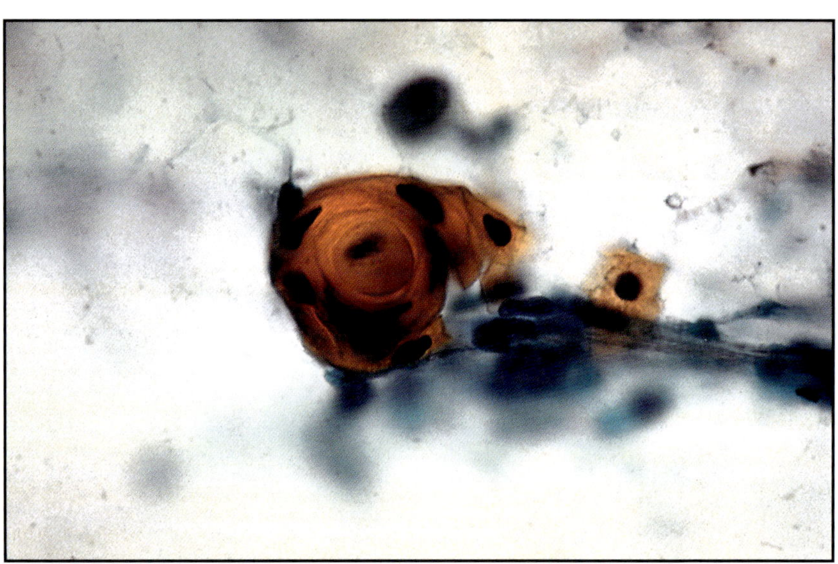

Image 5.38
Adenosquamous carcinoma of the endometrium. An epithelial pearl composed of malignant keratinizing squamous cells that have pyknotic nuclei and orangeophilic cytoplasm appears in a whorl arrangement (see Image 5.36). Endometrial brushing (Papanicolaou, 400X).

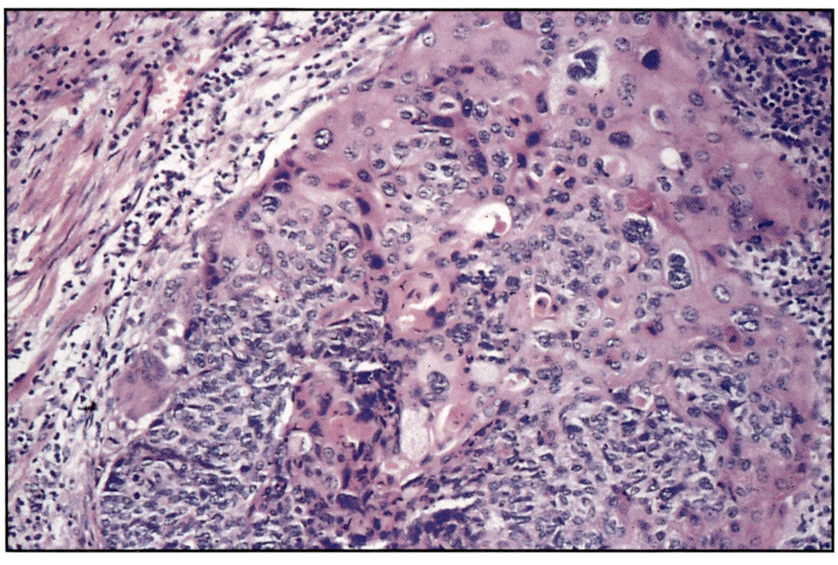

Image 5.39
Adenosquamous carcinoma of the endometrium. The tumor is characterized by a mixture of adenocarcinoma and keratinizing squamous cell carcinoma. The malignant glandular component is poorly differentiated. Histologic section (H&E, 100X).

Image 5.40
Clear cell carcinoma of the endometrium. The malignant cells have
large round nuclei with prominent
nuclei and an abundance of clear cytoplasm, and occur in three-dimensional,
cohesive groupings. Endometrial
brushing (Papanicolaou, 400X).

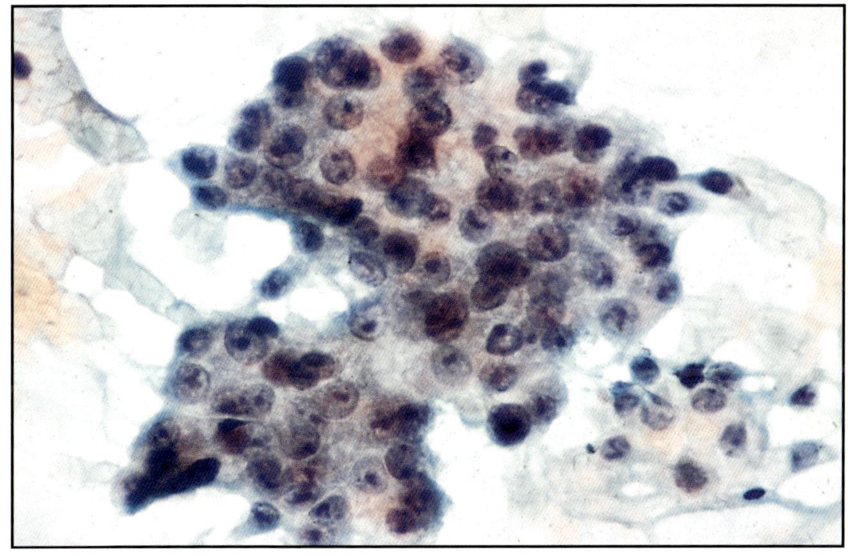

Image 5.41
Clear cell carcinoma of the endometrium. Large malignant cells have
large round nuclei and abundant clear
cytoplasm, and occur in acinar arrangements. Endometrial brushing (Papanicolaou, 400X).

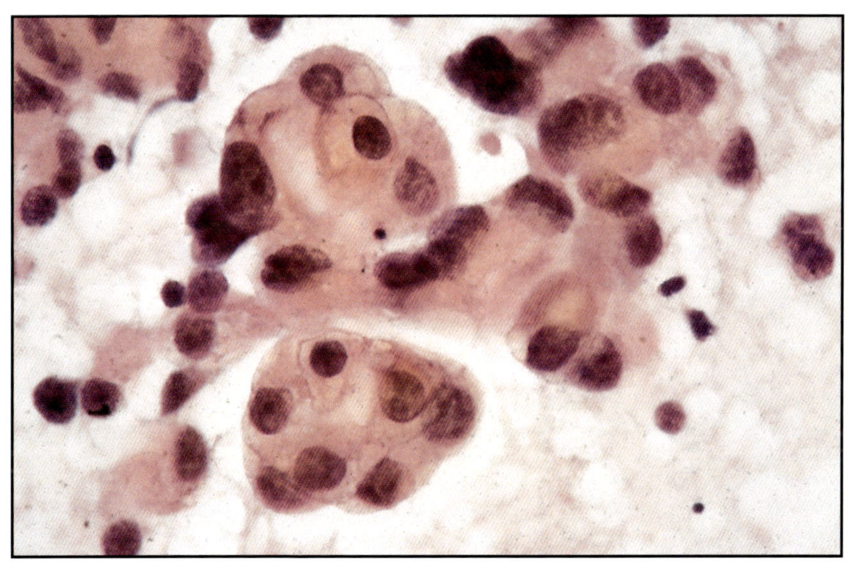

Image 5.42
Clear cell carcinoma of the endometrium. The tumor consists of solid
masses of large cells with abundant
clear cytoplasm and large round nuclei
with prominent nucleoli. Histologic
section (H&E, 100X).

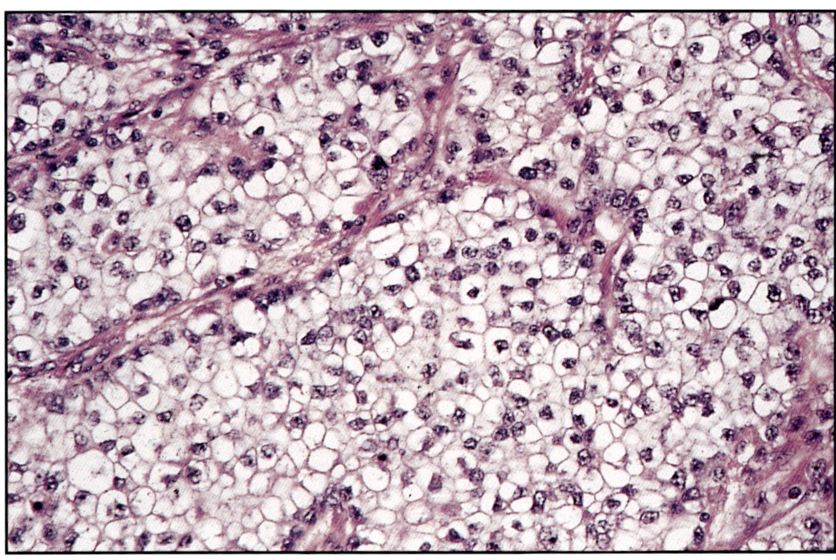

References

1. Alberhasky RC, Connelly PJ, Christopherson WM: Carcinoma of the endometrium: IV. Mixed adenosquamous carcinoma: A clinical-pathological study of 68 cases with long-term follow-up. *Am J Clin Pathol* 77:655–664, 1982.

2. Beckner ME, Mori T, Silverberg SG: Endometrial carcinoma: Non-tumor factors in prognosis. *Int J Gynecol Pathol* 4:131–145, 1985.

3. Berg JW, Lampe JG: High-risk factors in gynecologic cancer. *Cancer* 48:429–441, 1981.

4. Crum CP, Fechner RE: Clear cell adenocarcinoma of the endometrium: A clinicopathologic study of 11 cases. *Am J Diagn Gynecol Obstet* 1:261–267, 1979.

5. Deligdisch L, Cohen CJ: Histologic correlates and virulence implications of endometrial carcinoma associated with adenomatous hyperplasia. *Cancer* 56:1452–1455, 1985.

6. Deligdisch L, Holink CF: Progesterone receptors in two groups of endometrial carcinoma. *Cancer* 57:1385–1388, 1986.

7. Elwood MJ, Cole P, Rothman KJ, et al: Epidemiology of endometrial cancer. *J Natl Cancer Inst* 59:1055–1060, 1977.

8. Fox H, Sen DK: A controlled study of the constitutional stigmata of endometrial adenocarcinoma. *Br J Cancer* 24:30–36, 1970.

9. Geisinger KR, Marshall RB, Kute TE, et al: Correlation of female sex steroid hormone receptors with histologic and ultrastructural differentiation in adenocarcinoma of the endometrium. *Cancer* 58:1506–1517, 1986.

10. Judd HL, Davidson BJ, Frumar AM, et al: Serum androgens in postmenopausal women with and without endometrial cancer. *Am J Obstet Gynecol* 136:859–871, 1980.

11. Kurman RJ, Scully RE: Clear cell carcinoma of the endometrium: An analysis of 21 cases. *Cancer* 37:872–882, 1976.

12. Lynch HT, Krush AH, Larson AL: Heredity and endometrial carcinoma. *South Med J* 60:231, 1967.

13. Mack TM, Pike MC, Henderson BE, et al: Estrogens and endometrial cancer in a retirement community. *N Engl J Med* 294:1262–1267, 1976.

14. McCarty KS Jr, Barton TK, Peete CH Jr: Gonadal dysgenesis with adenocarcinoma of endometrium: An electron microscopic and steroid receptor analysis with a review of the literature. *Cancer* 42:512–520, 1978.

15. McDonald TW, Annegers JF, O'Dallon WM, et al: Exogenous estrogen and endometrial carcinoma: Case control and incidence study. *Am J Obstet Gynecol* 127:572–580, 1977.

16. McElin TW, Bird CC, Reeves BD, et al: Diagnostic dilation and curettages: A 20-year survey. *Obstet Gynecol* 33:807–812, 1969.

17. Musubuchi K, Nemoto H: Epidemiologic studies on uterine cancer at Cancer Institute Hospital, Tokyo, Japan. *Cancer* 30:268–275, 1972.

18. Ng ABP, Reagan JW, Storaasli JP, et al: Mixed adenosquamous carcinoma of the endometrium. *Am J Clin Pathol* 59:765–781, 1973.

19. Pacheco JC, Kempers RD: Etiology of postmenopausal bleeding. *Obstet Gynecol* 32:40–46, 1968.

20. Pertschuk LP, Beddoe AM, Gorelic LS, et al: Immunocytochemical assay of estrogen receptors in endometrial carcinoma with monoclonal antibodies: Comparison with biochemical assay. *Cancer* 57:1000–1004, 1986.

21. Pfleider A, Kleine W: Risk factors of endometrial carcinoma. In: *Endometrial Cancers,* Bolla M, Racinet C, Vrousos C (editors). New York, NY, S Karger, 1986, p 12.

22. Robboy SJ, Bradley R: Changing trends and prognostic features in endometrial cancer associated with exogenous estrogen therapy. *Obstet Gynecol* 54:269–277, 1979.

23. Robboy SJ, Miller AW III, Kurman RJ: The pathologic features and behavior of endometrial carcinoma associated with exogenous estrogen administration. *Pathol Res Pract* 174:237–256, 1982.

24. Rosai J: *Ackerman's Surgical Pathology.* 7th ed. St Louis, MO, CV Mosby Co, 1989, pp 1050–1097.

25. Salazar OM, DePapp EW, Bonfiglio TA, et al: Adenosquamous carcinoma of the endometrium: An entity with an inherently poor prognosis? *Cancer* 40:119–130, 1977.

26. Shapiro S, Kelly JP, Rosenberg L, et al: Risk of localized and widespread endometrial cancer in relation to recent and discontinued use of conjugated estrogen. *N Engl J Med* 313:969–972, 1985.

27. Siiteri PK: Steroid hormones and endometrial cancer. *Cancer Res* 38:4360–4366, 1978.

28. Silverberg SG, Bolin MG, De Giorgi LS: Adenoacanthoma and mixed adenosquamous carcinoma of the endometrium: A clinicopathologic study. *Cancer* 30:1307–1314, 1972.

29. Silverberg SG, Makowski EL, Roche WD: Endometrial carcinoma in women under 40 years of age. *Cancer* 39:592–598, 1977.

30. Silverberg SG, Mullen D, Faraci JA, et al: Endometrial carcinoma: Clinical-pathologic comparison of cases in postmenopausal women receiving and not receiving exogenous estrogens. *Cancer* 45:3018–3026, 1980.

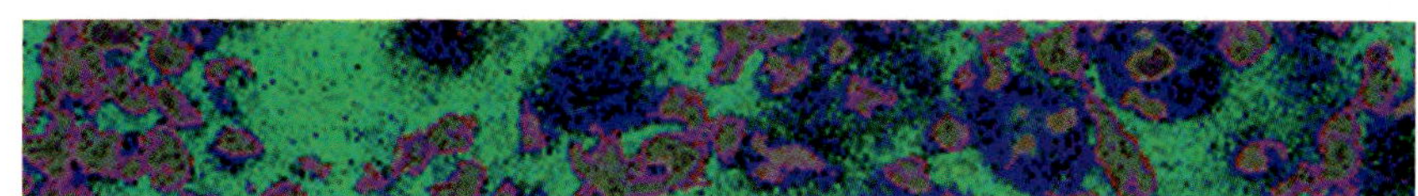

CHAPTER SIX

Uterine Sarcoma

Uterine sarcomas represent 3% of malignant uterine corporeal tumors. Their clinical presentation is essentially identical to that of endometrial carcinoma; however, the history of hyperestrogenism and the clinical triad of obesity, hypertension, and diabetes often seen in women with endometrial carcinoma are of less significance to the diagnosis of sarcomas. Uterine sarcomas are of mesodermal origin. In our practical work, endometrial stromal sarcoma, leiomyosarcoma, and mixed müllerian tumors are occasionally encountered; other sarcomas are extremely rare.

Endometrial Stromal Sarcoma

Endometrial stromal sarcomas tend to occur in middle-aged women. More than one half of the patients are premenopausal; rarely does stromal sarcoma occur in young women.[3,5] There is no association with endometrial carcinoma risk factors, but a few patients have a history of prior pelvic irradiation.[1]

Endometrial stromal sarcomas have two forms: low-grade and high-grade.[4,11] They are composed of cells resembling the stromal cells of proliferating endometrium.

Low-Grade Stromal Sarcoma

Low-grade stromal sarcoma invades the myometrium and may extensively permeate it. Invasion of lymphatic and vascular channels is also common. The tumors are usually slow-growing, and recurrences are commonly detected many years after initial treatment. The cells in a low-grade stromal sarcoma show little nuclear variation and have ovoid nuclei with dispersed, slightly coarse chromatin and small or inconspicuous nucleoli. The cytoplasm is ill-defined. The uniformity of the cells imparts a monotonous appearance. Mitotic figures are increased, but these are usually fewer than nine per ten high-power fields. A prominent vascular pattern is frequently present.

In endometrial brushing preparations from low-grade stromal sarcomas, numerous tumor cells lie singly, with some loose groups and a few cohesive groupings of tumor cells. Very few glandular cells are seen in the brushing preparations. The tumor cells have relatively uniform and regular, ovoid nuclei with slightly coarse chromatin and inconspicuous nucleoli. The average nuclear size is larger than that of normal stromal cells. The cytoplasm is scant and often ill-defined, appearing as many stripped nuclei (Images 6.1–6.4). Although the tumor cells of low-grade stromal sarcoma are somewhat benign-looking, the presence of a large number of solitary stromal cells with enlarged nuclei and the lack of glandular cells in a direct endometrial sample are important clues to the cytologic diagnosis of low-grade stromal sarcoma.

High-Grade Stromal Sarcoma

High-grade stromal sarcomas often infiltrate the myometrium destructively, with necrosis. The tumors are characterized by rapid progression. They are composed of cells that are usually considerably more atypical than those in low-grade stromal sarcomas. The tumors have ten or more mitotic figures per ten high-power fields. Recurrences are common and are usually evident within 2 years after the initial treatment.

In endometrial brushing preparations from high-grade stromal sarcomas, the tumor cells usually lie singly and show variations in nuclear size and shape. Their nuclei are enlarged, and have coarsely granular chromatin and frequent prominent nucleoli. Multinucleated tumor cells are present. The cytoplasm is scant and ill-defined, given the appearance of many stripped nuclei (Images 6.5–6.8). The cytologic diagnosis of high-grade stromal sarcomas, unlike that of low-grade tumors, is usually straightforward.

Leiomyosarcoma

Leiomyosarcoma accounts for about 1.3% of uterine malignancy and about 25% of uterine sarcomas. They occur in an older age group; the mean age of patients is 52 years, nearly a decade older than the mean age of patients with leiomyomas. Most leiomyosarcomas are solitary masses within the uterus. They are soft and fleshy, with areas of necrosis and hemorrhage. Histologically, they are composed of round, ovoid to spindle cells with the morphologic, ultrastructural, and immunocytochemical features of smooth muscle cells. Actin and desmin are consistently present in their cytoplasm, and can be demonstrated by immunoperoxidase stainings. On the basis of cytomorphologic features of smooth muscle tumors in correlation with histology, the malignant ones can be classified into low-grade leiomyosarcoma, high-grade leiomyosarcoma, and malignant leiomyoblastoma.

Low-Grade Leiomyosarcoma

In endometrial brushing preparations, the tumor cells occur singly, in loose groupings, or in closely packed, cohesive groupings. They have ovoid, spindle-shaped, or elongated nuclei, some of which are very long (cigar-shaped) with blunt ends. The cigar-shaped nuclei with a finely or slightly coarsely granular chromatin pattern are often in parallel, side-by-side arrangements. Their cytoplasm is scant and ill-defined. Some of the tumor cells appear as many stripped nuclei, and others exhibit extended, bipolar cytoplasmic processes (Images 6.9–6.12). Multinucleated tumor cells are infrequently encountered in low-grade tumors.

High-Grade Leiomyosarcoma

In endometrial brushing preparations, the tumor cells lie singly or occur in loose groupings. They have ovoid, elongated or irregular-shaped nuclei with coarse clumping of chromatin. Pleomorphism of the nuclei is apparent. The tumor cells have very scant, ill-defined cytoplasm. In fact, many of them have no recognizable cytoplasm, appearing as stripped nuclei. Frequent multinucleation is noted, and the multinucleated tumor cells often have a small to moderate amount of cytoplasm (Images 6.13–6.17). Mitotic figures are frequently found. Necrotic tumor debris is often seen.

Malignant Leiomyoblastoma

Occasional leiomyosarcomas of the uterus have an epithelioid appearance and are referred to as malignant leiomyoblastomas. In endometrial brushing preparations, tumor cells lie singly or occur in loose groupings or rarely in cohesive groupings. They have round or ovoid nuclei with a coarsely granular chromatin pattern. Small nucleoli are seen in some of the tumor cells. There is an apparent variation in nuclear size. The tumor cells have scant, ill-defined cytoplasm or no recognizable cytoplasm, appearing as many stripped nuclei. Multinucleated tumor cells are not seen (Images 6.18–6.20).

Cytologic Differentiation Between Low-Grade Leiomyosarcoma and Leiomyoma

In histologic diagnosis of smooth muscle tumors, the single most important criterion for distinguishing a leiomyosarcoma from a leiomyoma is the number of mitotic figures present. As a rule, a smooth muscle tumor that has more than five mitoses per ten high-power fields is considered to be malignant.[2,10] Tumors with ten or more mitoses per ten high-power fields behave almost always as malignant neoplasms, even if atypia is minimal.[7] For epithelioid smooth muscle tumors (leiomyoblastomas), a finding of more than five mitoses per 50 high-power fields is considered to be malignant.[2] In cytologic diagnosis of smooth muscle

Table 6.1
The Cytologic Differentiation Between
Low-Grade Leiomyosarcoma and Leiomyoma

Cytologic Findings	Low-Grade Leiomyosarcoma	Leiomyoma
Cellular arrangements	Closely packed cohesive groupings, loose groupings, numerous solitary cells; tumor cells in parallel arrangements	Mainly cohesive groupings with a syncytial appearance
Nuclear shape	Ovoid, spindle-shaped, or cigar-shaped with blunt ends	Ovoid, spindle-shaped, or elongated
Multinucleation	Present	Absent
Amount of cytoplasm	Scanty or appearing as stripped nuclei	Abundant with ill-defined cell borders
Vascularity	Blood vessels seen in tumor fragments	No blood vessels seen
Necrosis	May be present	Usually absent

tumors, this criterion cannot be used for the cytologic differentiation between malignant and benign neoplasms due to the sampling problem in a small amount of specimen.[9] It is not uncommon that mitotic figures are absent in cytologic preparations from low-grade leiomyosarcomas.[9] In brushing preparations from high-grade leiomyosarcoma, the mitotic figure rate cannot easily be compared from one case to another.

However, mitotic count in uterine smooth muscle tumors has been criticized because of its apparent lack of standardization and reproducibility.[8] The number of mitotic figures can be influenced by the thickness of the histologic section, tumor sampling, discrepancy among examiners, microscopic magnification, and uneven distribution of mitotic figures in tumors.

Having considered the problems in histologic diagnosis of smooth muscle tumors and the sampling problem for mitotic figures in cytologic preparations, we consider the cytomorphologic features that are helpful in differentiating a leiomyosarcoma from a leiomyoma.[9] Although the histologic differentiation between low-grade leiomyosarcoma and leiomyoma is sometimes difficult, on the basis of the cytomorphologic features of various types of smooth muscle tumors, it appears possible to distinguish a low-grade leiomyosarcoma from a leiomyoma.[9] The cytologic criteria that are helpful in the differentiation between low-grade leiomyosarcoma and leiomyoma[9] are elucidated in Table 6.1. In the cytologic diagnosis of high-grade leiomyosarcoma, the cytomorphologic features, such as pleomorphism of tumor cells, low intercellular cohesion, frequent multinucleation, and high mitotic rate, coupled with immunoperoxidase stainings (for actin and desmin), do not present any differential diagnostic problem.

Mixed Müllerian Tumor

Mixed müllerian tumors (mixed mesodermal tumors) are rare uterine neoplasms that are seen almost solely in postmenopausal patients (mean age,

65 years). They usually arise in the uterine body, the most common site being the posterior wall in the region of the fundus. They present as large, soft, polypoid growths involving the endometrium and myometrium. Infertility, obesity, diabetes, and hypertension also occur in patients with mixed müllerian tumor, but their association with mixed müllerian tumor is not as clear as it is with endometrial carcinoma. A few patients have a history of pelvic irradiation.[1] The depth of myometrial invasion rather than morphologic features of a mixed müllerian tumor has prognostic value.

Microscopically, the characteristic feature of mixed müllerian tumor is the admixture of carcinomatous and sarcomatous elements, with the latter usually predominating. However, there are also tumors, especially metastatic tumors, in which the malignant stroma is so inconspicuous as to be missed altogether; as a result, the tumors are often misdiagnosed as an adenocarcinoma. The carcinomatous component is typically an adenocarcinoma of the endometrioid type. In 5% of mixed müllerian tumors, the epithelial component is squamous carcinoma. The appearance of the sarcomatous component is the basis for the division of these tumors into a homologous and a heterologous variety.[4–6] The distinction between these two varieties may not be possible if the endometrial brushing preparation is scantily cellular.

Homologous Mixed Müllerian Tumor

In homologous mixed müllerian tumor (carcinosarcoma), the most common sarcomatous components are fibrosarcoma and endometrial stromal sarcoma. Leiomyosarcoma is less frequent. Mixtures of fibrosarcoma, leiomyosarcoma, and/or stromal sarcoma also occur.

In endometrial brushing preparations from homologous mixed müllerian tumors, a few groups of adenocarcinoma cells intermix with either spindle tumor cells resembling fibrosarcoma or leiomyosarcoma, or ovoid tumor cells resembling stromal sarcoma. Sarcomatous components are usually predominant (Images 6.21–6.24). Rarely, malignant squamous cells are encountered.

Heterologous Mixed Müllerian Tumor

In this variety, heterologous components tend to be found in association with areas of undifferentiated sarcoma or high-grade stromal sarcoma. Skeletal muscle and/or rhabdomyosarcoma is the most common heterologous element. Cartilage is the second most common heterologous element. Less common heterologous elements include osseous tissue and fat.

In endometrial brushing preparations from heterologous mixed müllerian tumors, heterologous mesenchymal elements, such as skeletal muscle, cartilage, osseous tissue, and/or fat, are present in association with adenocarcinoma cells and sarcomatous tumor cells, which are usually undifferentiated or resemble high-grade stromal sarcoma. Specific heterologous mesenchymal elements and sarcomatous components usually predominate (Images 6.25–6.32). Pure and mixed heterologous endometrial sarcomas occur very rarely. They differ from heterologous mixed müllerian tumors by the absence of an epithelial component.

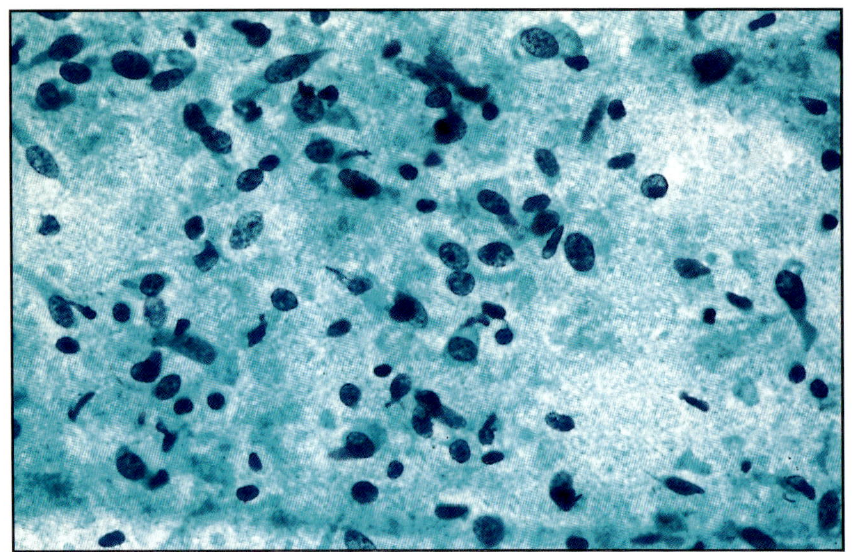

Image 6.1
Low-grade stromal sarcoma of the uterus. The malignant cells have large, relatively uniform and regular, ovoid nuclei with slightly coarsely granular chromatin and inconspicuous nucleoli, and scant, ill-defined cytoplasm. They occur as solitary cells. Endometrial brushing (Papanicolaou, 200X).

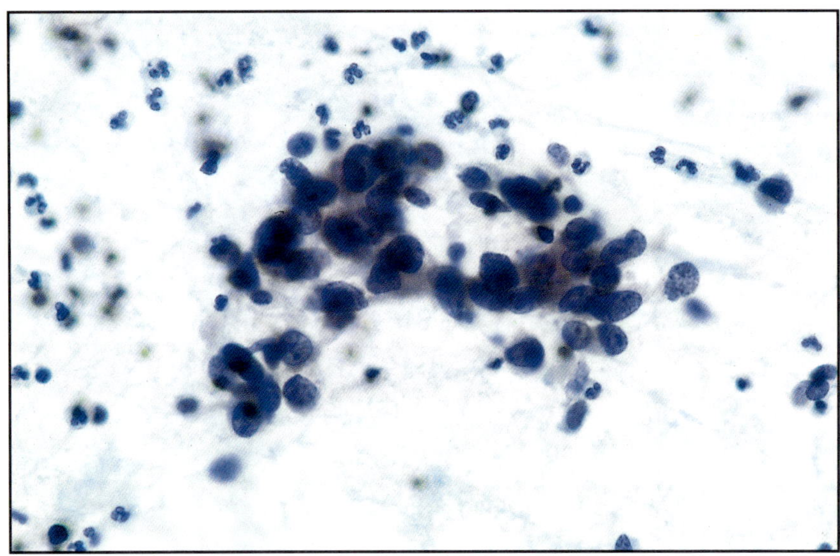

Image 6.2
Low-grade stromal sarcoma of the uterus. The malignant cells have ovoid nuclei with slightly coarse chromatin and very scant, ill-defined cytoplasm, appearing as many stripped nuclei. They occur in loose groupings. Endometrial brushing (Papanicolaou, 400X).

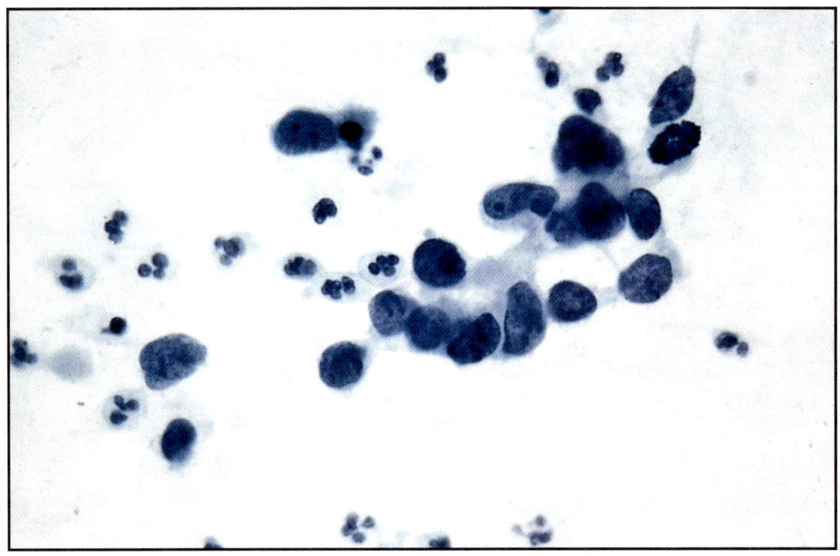

Image 6.3
Low-grade stromal sarcoma of the uterus. The malignant cells appear as many stripped nuclei and show some variations in nuclear size and shape. Note that occasional mitotic figures are present. Endometrial brushing (Papanicolaou, 400X).

Image 6.4
Low-grade stromal sarcoma of the
uterus. The tumor is composed of
masses of cells resembling endometrial
stromal cells that have ovoid nuclei with
dispersed chromatin and inconspicuous
nucleoli. Mitotic figures are increased.
Histologic section (H&E, 100X).

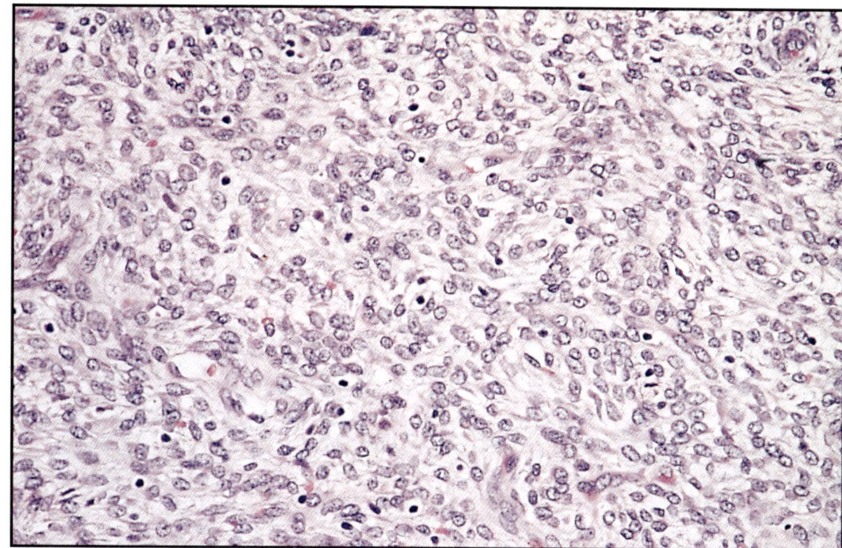

Image 6.5
High-grade stromal sarcoma of the
uterus. The malignant cells have large,
pleomorphic nuclei with coarse chromatin and very scant, ill-defined cytoplasm, and occur in loose groupings or
as solitary cells. Note that mitotic figures
are present. Endometrial brushing (Papanicolaou, 400X).

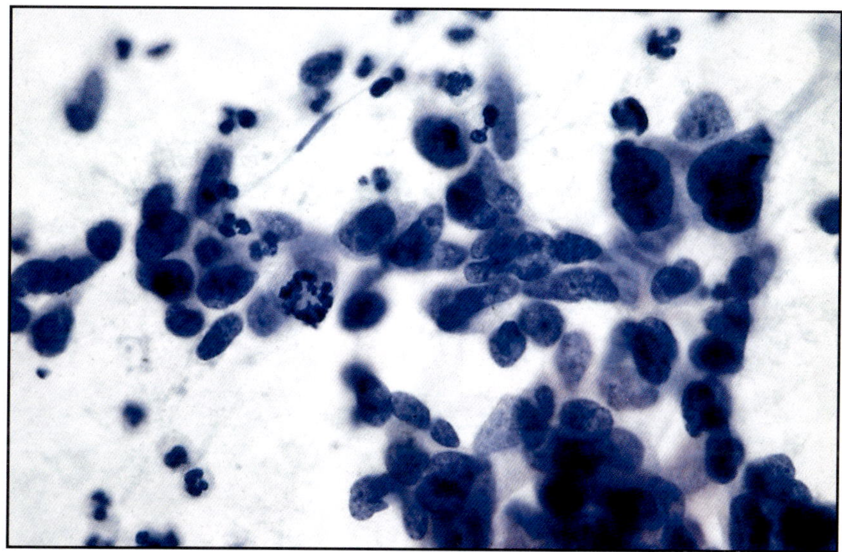

Image 6.6
High-grade stromal sarcoma of the
uterus. The malignant cells have large,
pleomorphic nuclei with slightly coarse
chromatin and prominent nucleoli, and
scant, ill-defined cytoplasm. They
occur as solitary cells. Endometrial
brushing (Papanicolaou, 400X).

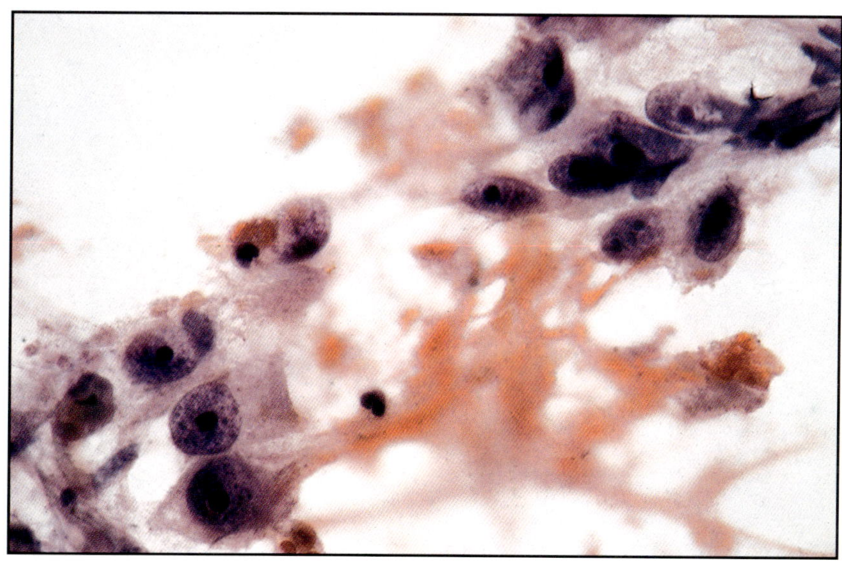

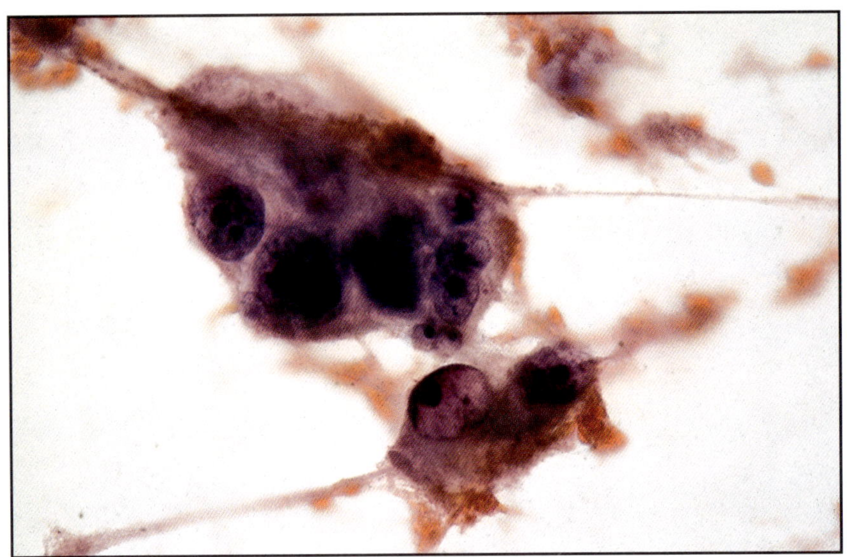

Image 6.7
High-grade stromal sarcoma of the uterus. A giant malignant cell has several pleomorphic nuclei with prominent nucleoli and lightly stained cytoplasm. Endometrial brushing (Papanicolaou, 400X).

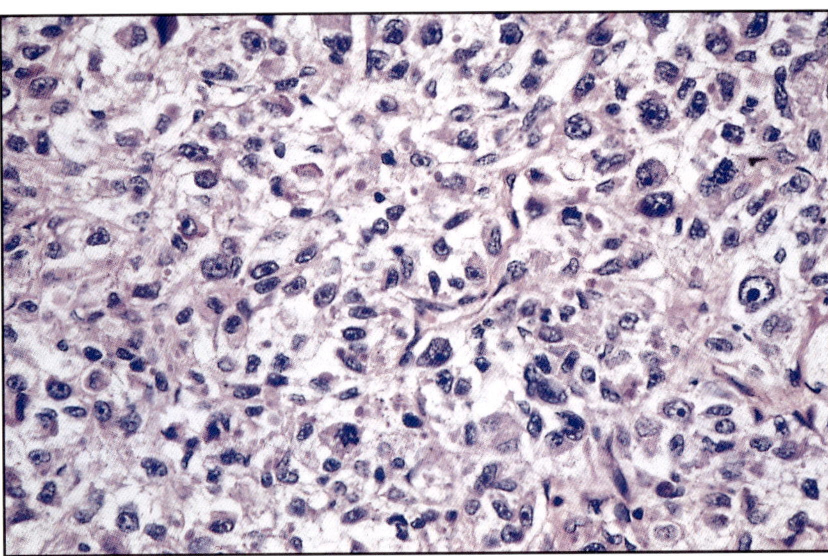

Image 6.8
High-grade stromal sarcoma of the uterus. The tumor is composed of cells that are considerably more atypical than those shown in Image 6.4. The tumor cells have large, pleomorphic nuclei with prominent nucleoli, and have frequent mitotic figures. Histologic section (H&E, 200X).

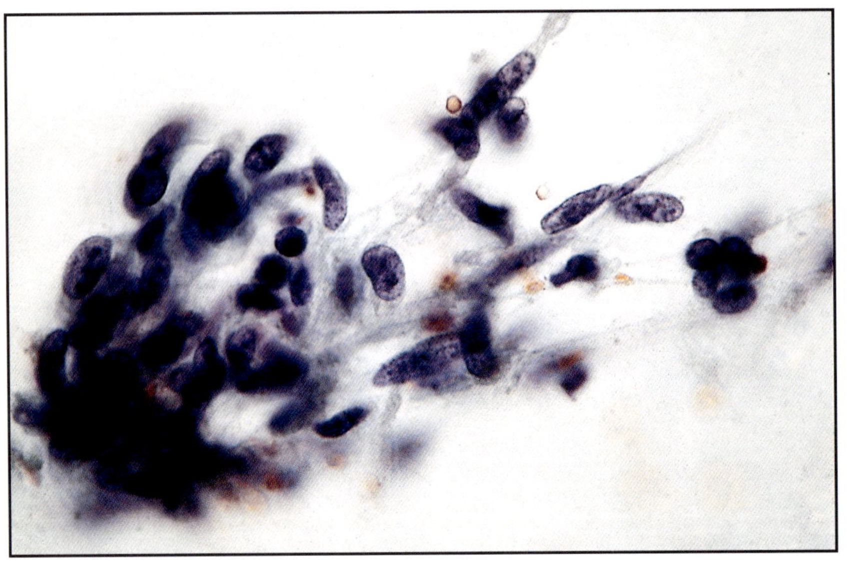

Image 6.9
Low-grade leiomyosarcoma of the uterus. The malignant cells have ovoid, fusiform, or elongated nuclei with finely granular chromatin and scant, ill-defined cytoplasm. They occur in loose groupings. Endometrial brushing (Papanicolaou, 400X).

Image 6.10
Low-grade leiomyosarcoma of the uterus. The malignant cells have cigar-shaped nuclei with blunt ends. Some of them appear as stripped nuclei and others show extended, bipolar cytoplasmic processes. Endometrial brushing (Papanicolaou, 400X).

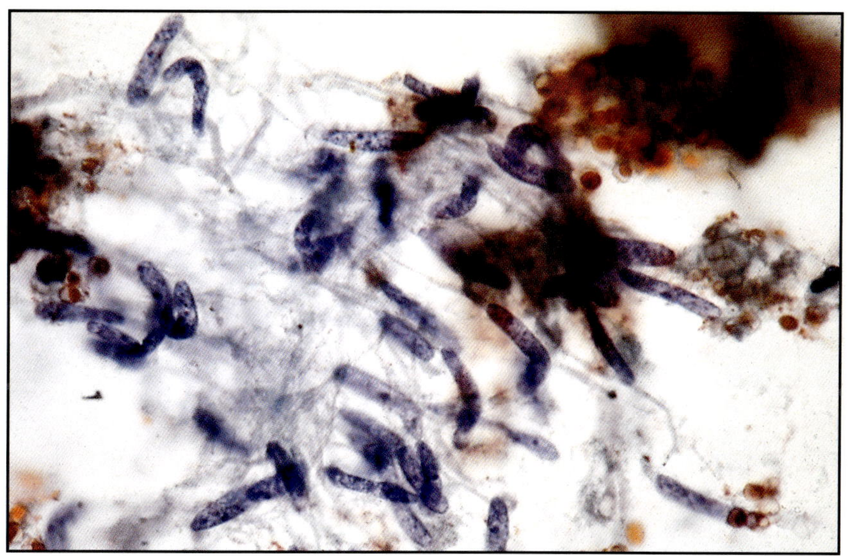

Image 6.11
Low-grade leiomyosarcoma of the uterus. The malignant cells have cigar-shaped nuclei and ill-defined cytoplasm, and occur in a parallel, side-by-side arrangement. Endometrial brushing (Papanicolaou, 400X).

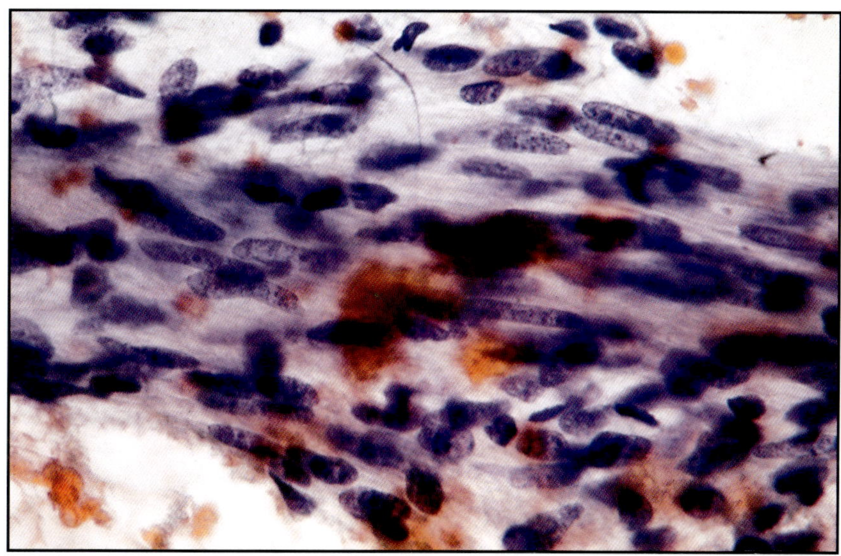

Image 6.12
Low-grade leiomyosarcoma of the uterus. The tumor is composed of bundles of spindle cells with fusiform or cigar-shaped nuclei. Frequent mitotic figures are noticed. Histologic section (H&E, 200X).

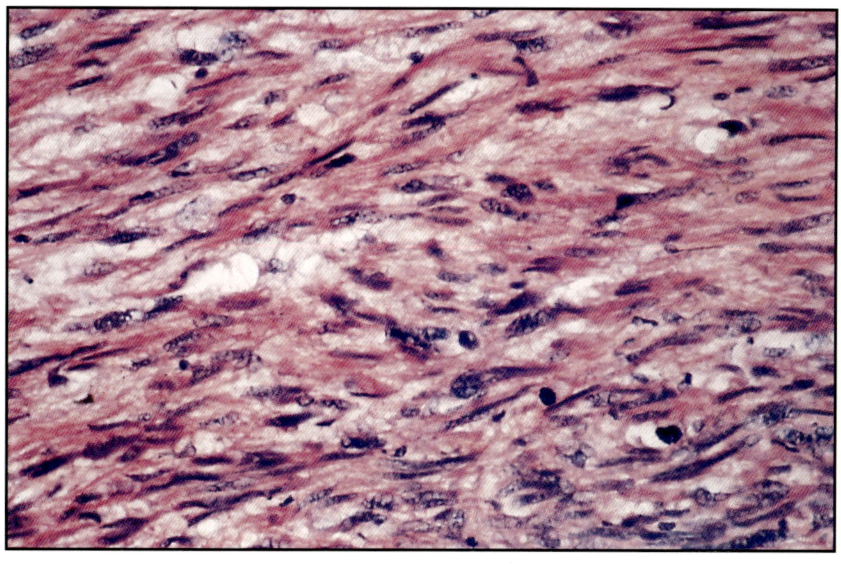

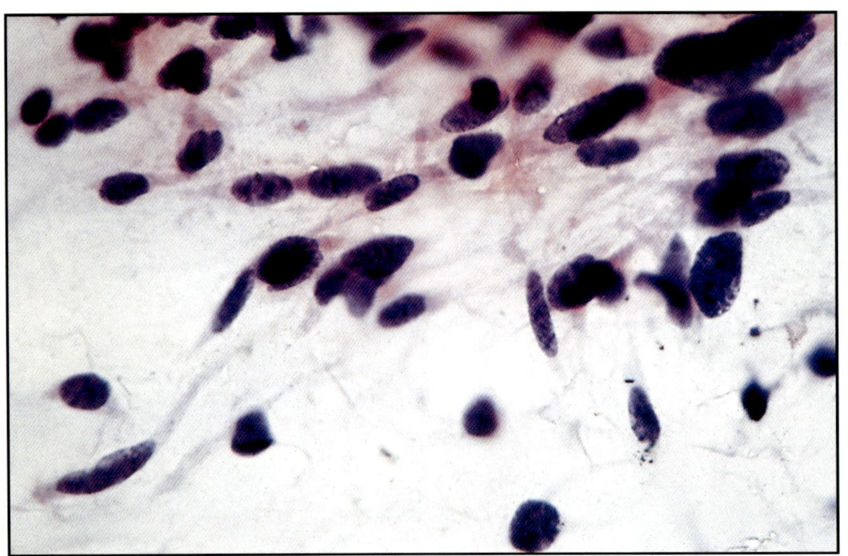

Image 6.13
High-grade leiomyosarcoma of the uterus. The malignant cells have ovoid, elongated, or irregular-shaped nuclei with coarse chromatin and scant, ill-defined cytoplasm. They occur in loose groupings or as solitary cells. Endometrial brushing (Papanicolaou, 400X).

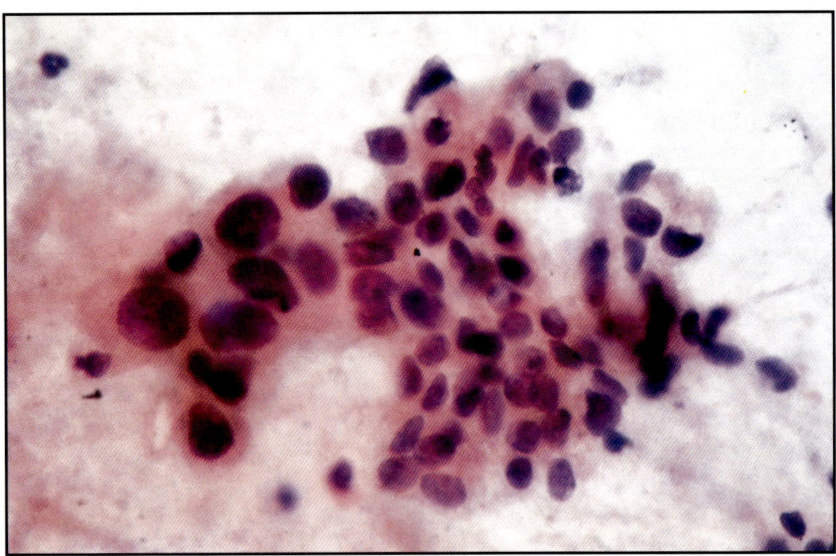

Image 6.14
High-grade leiomyosarcoma of the uterus. The malignant cells have pleomorphic nuclei that show marked variations in nuclear size and shape and have coarse chromatin. Endometrial brushing (Papanicolaou, 400X).

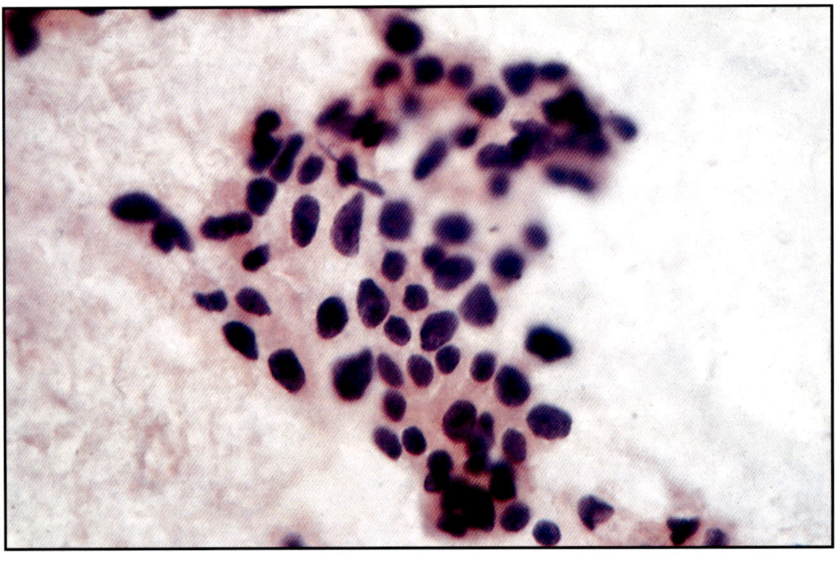

Image 6.15
High-grade leiomyosarcoma of the uterus. The malignant cells have hyperchromatic nuclei with coarse chromatin and little recognizable cytoplasm, appearing as many stripped nuclei. Endometrial brushing (Papanicolaou, 400X).

Image 6.16
High-grade leiomyosarcoma of the
uterus. A giant malignant cell has several
nuclei with coarse clumping of chromatin and a small amount of ill-defined
cytoplasm. Note that the nuclei show a
variation in size. Endometrial brushing
(Papanicolaou, 400X).

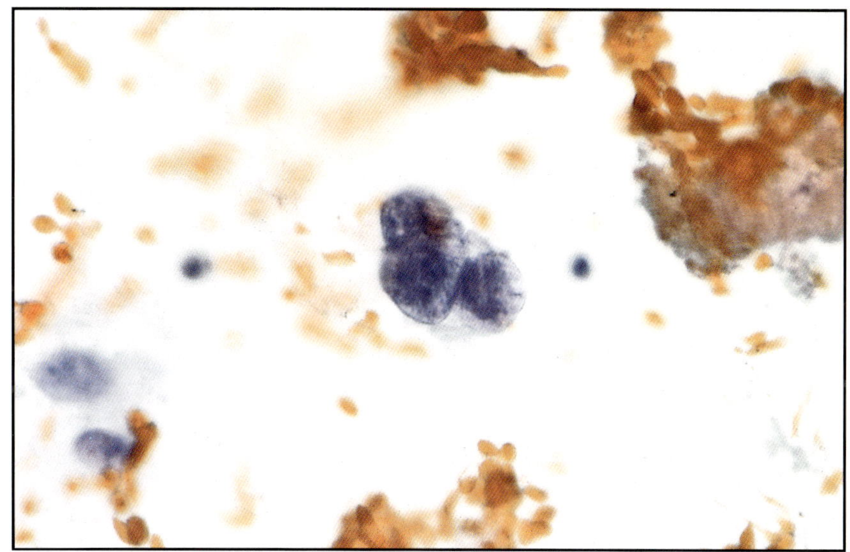

Image 6.17
High-grade leiomyosarcoma of the
uterus. The tumor is composed of cells
that are considerably more atypical
than those shown in Image 6.12.
Mitotic figures are also more frequent,
and multinucleated tumor cells are
noted. Histologic section (H&E, 200X).

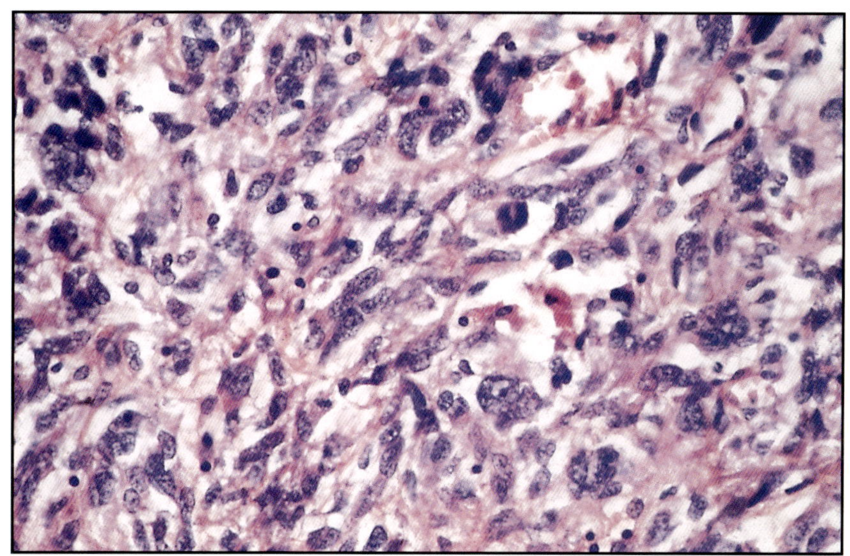

Image 6.18
Malignant leiomyoblastoma of the
uterus. The malignant cells have round
or ovoid nuclei with coarse chromatin
and scant, ill-defined cytoplasm, and
occur as solitary cells. Endometrial
brushing (Papanicolaou, 400X).

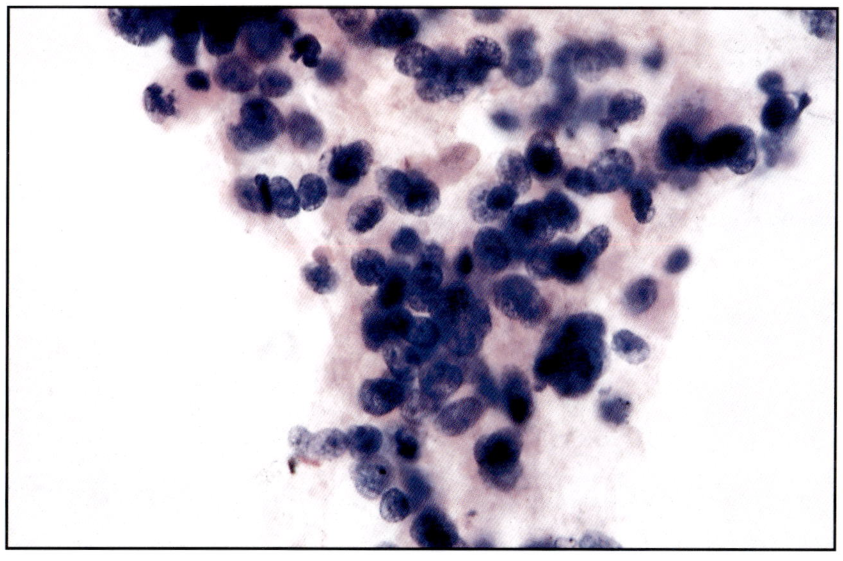

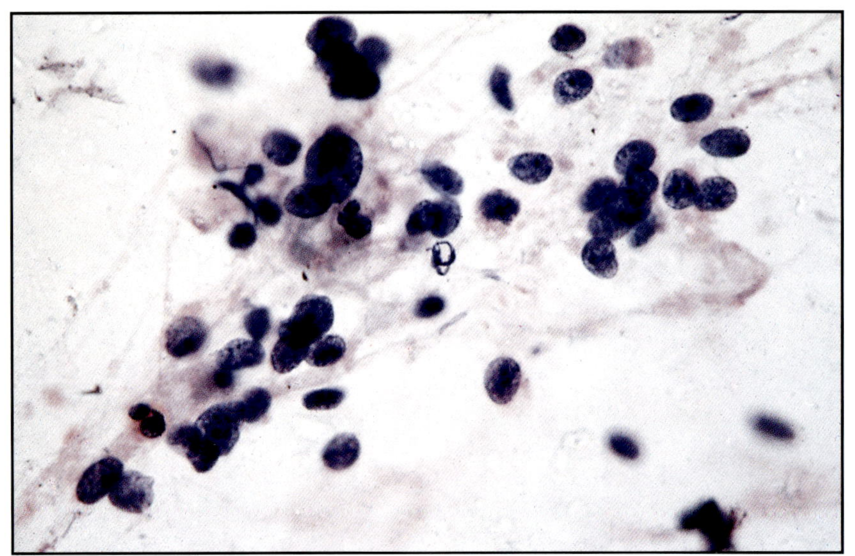

Image 6.19
Malignant leiomyoblastoma of the uterus. The malignant cells have hyperchromatic nuclei with occasional small nucleoli and variation in nuclear size. Their cytoplasm is not recognizable, appearing as many stripped nuclei. Endometrial brushing (Papanicolaou, 400X).

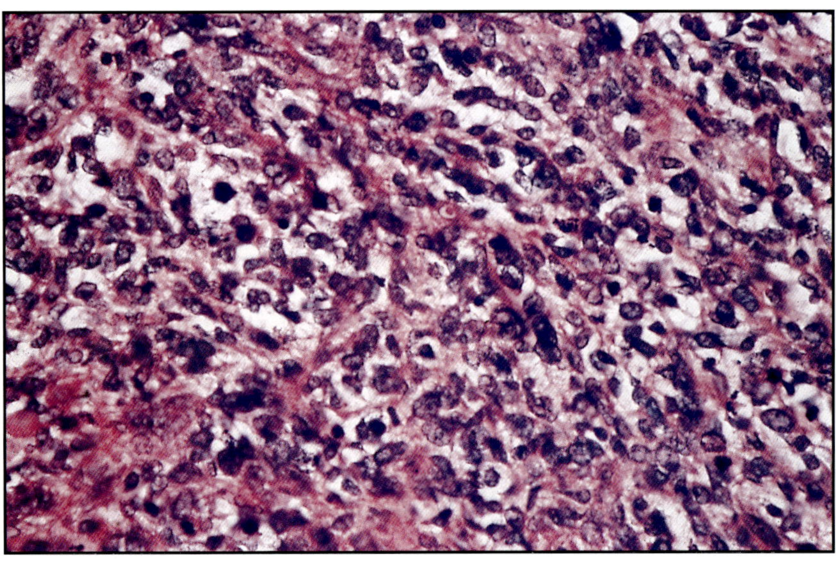

Image 6.20
Malignant leiomyoblastoma of the uterus. The tumor is composed of masses of cells that have an epithelioid appearance. The tumor cells have round or ovoid nuclei and are disorderly arranged. Histologic section (H&E, 200X).

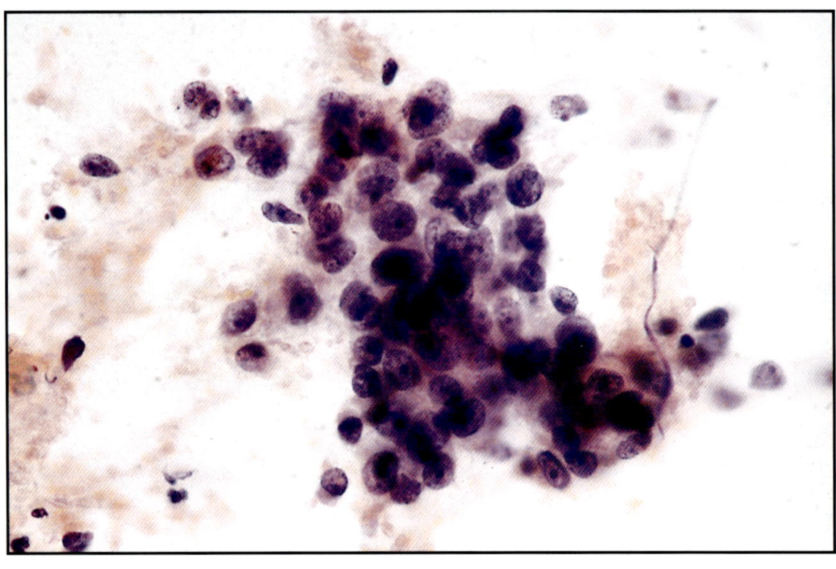

Image 6.21
Homologous mixed müllerian tumor of the uterus. Loose groups of malignant cells that have large, round or ovoid nuclei with slightly coarse chromatin and occasional prominent nuclei and scant, ill-defined cytoplasm resemble moderately differentiated endometrial adenocarcinoma (see Images 6.22 and 6.23). Endometrial brushing (Papanicolaou, 400X).

Image 6.22
Homologous mixed müllerian tumor
of the uterus. Loose groups of malignant cells that have ovoid nuclei with
slightly coarse chromatin and inconspicuous nucleoli and scant, ill-defined
cytoplasm resemble uterine stromal sarcoma (see Image 6.21). Endometrial
brushing (Papanicolaou, 400X).

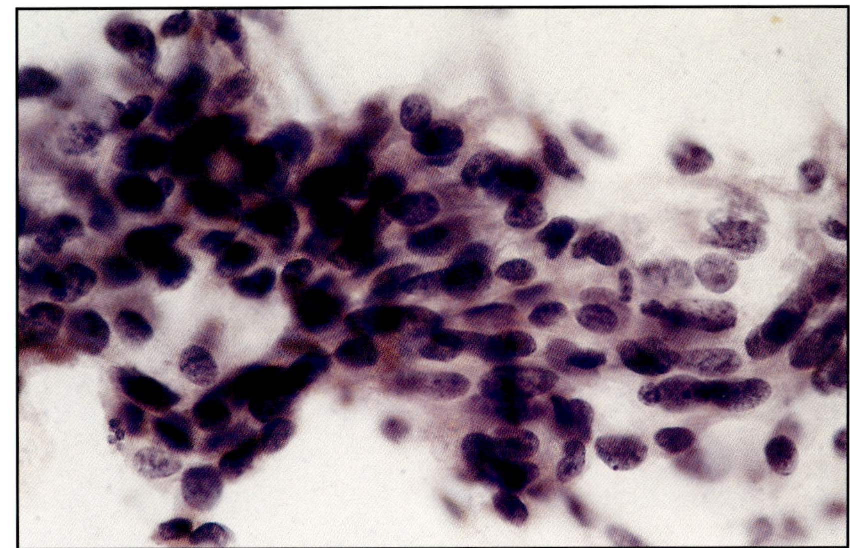

Image 6.23
Homologous mixed müllerian tumor
of the uterus. The malignant cells have
ovoid nuclei with slightly coarse chromatin and small nucleoli, and little
recognizable cytoplasm, appearing as
many stripped nuclei. These features
are consistent with uterine stromal sarcoma (see Image 6.21). Endometrial
brushing (Papanicolaou, 400X).

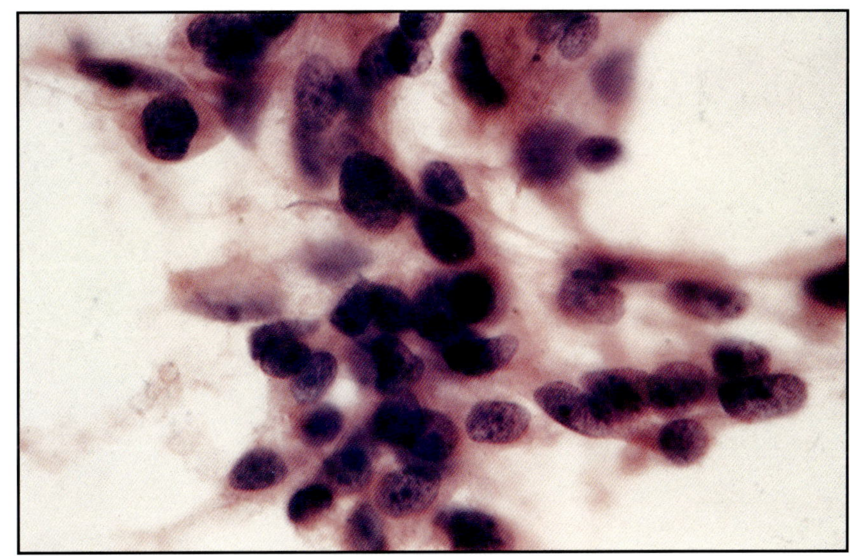

Image 6.24
Homologous mixed müllerian tumor of
the uterus. The tumor is characterized
by the admixture of carcinomatous and
sarcomatous elements. The carcinomatous element is an adenocarcinoma of
the endometrioid type (see Image
6.21), and the sarcomatous element
resembles stromal sarcoma of the uterus
(see Images 6.22 and 6.23). Histologic
section (H&E, 100X).

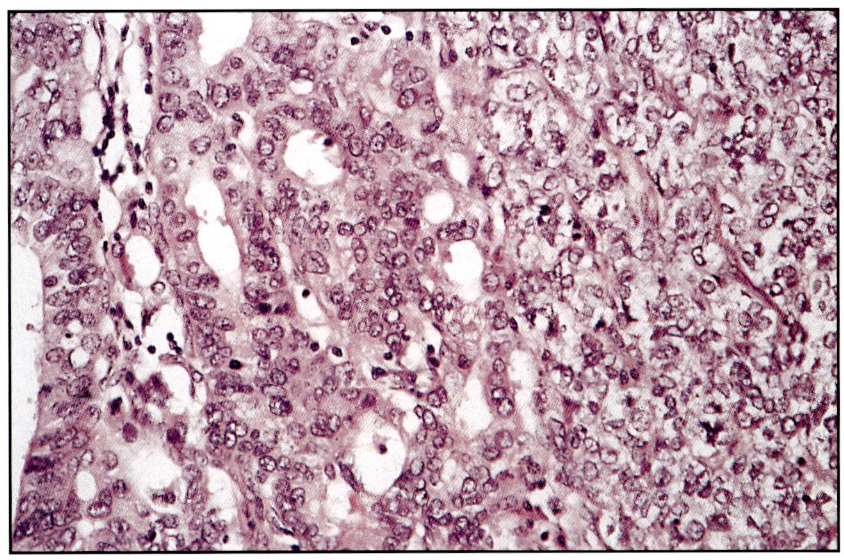

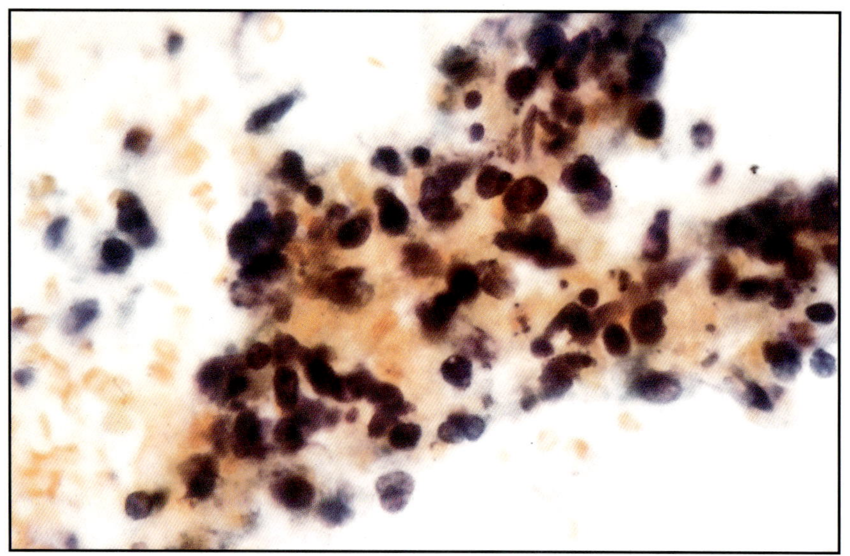

Image 6.25
Heterologous mixed müllerian tumor of the uterus. The malignant cells have hyperchromatic nuclei with coarse chromatin and little recognizable cytoplasm and show marked variations in nuclear size and shape. These features resemble those of high-grade uterine stromal sarcoma. Other components are shown in Images 6.26-6.30. Endometrial brushing (Papanicolaou, 400X).

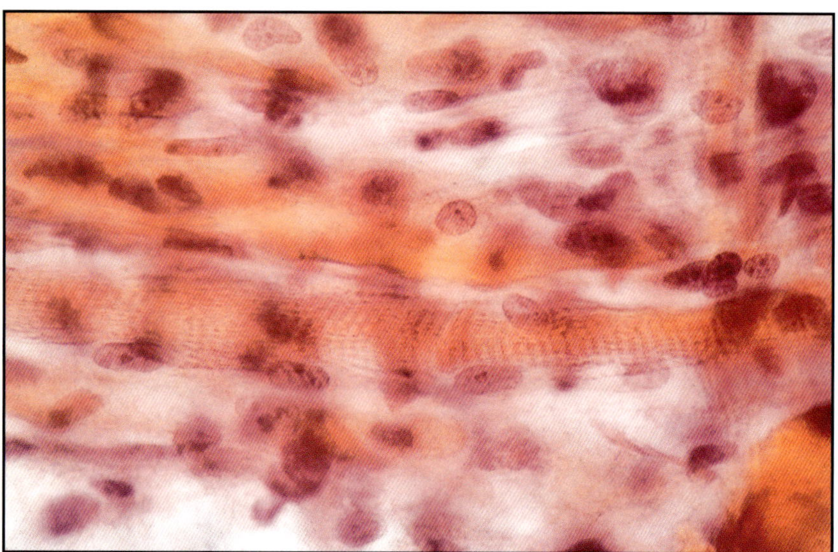

Image 6.26
Heterologous mixed müllerian tumor of the uterus. The tumor shows skeletal muscle differentiation. A striated muscle cell with cross striations is identified (see Image 6.25). Endometrial brushing (Papanicolaou, 200X).

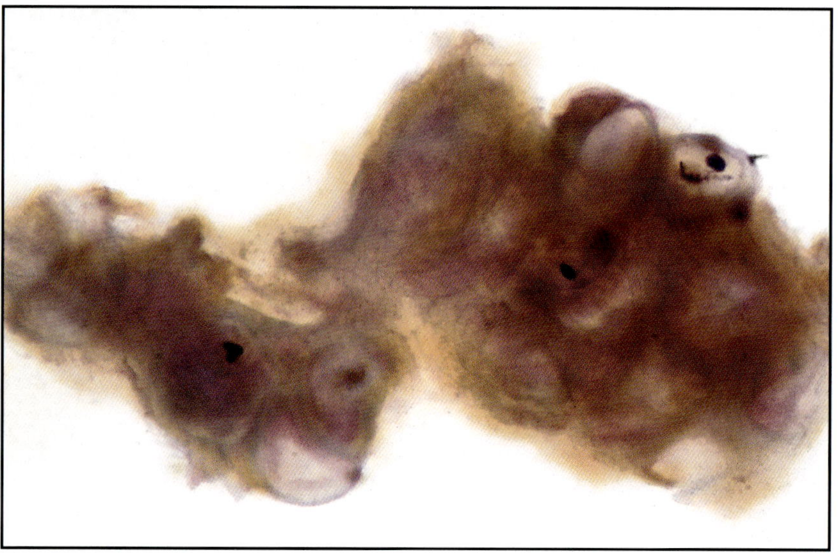

Image 6.27
Heterologous mixed müllerian tumor of the uterus. A fragment of cartilage contains abundant cartilaginous matrix and a few chondrocytes (see Image 6.25). Endometrial brushing (Papanicolaou, 100X).

Image 6.28
Heterologous mixed müllerian tumor
of the uterus. Two chondrocytes are
surrounded by a ring of cartilaginous
matrix (see Image 6.25). Endometrial
brushing (Papanicolaou, 200X).

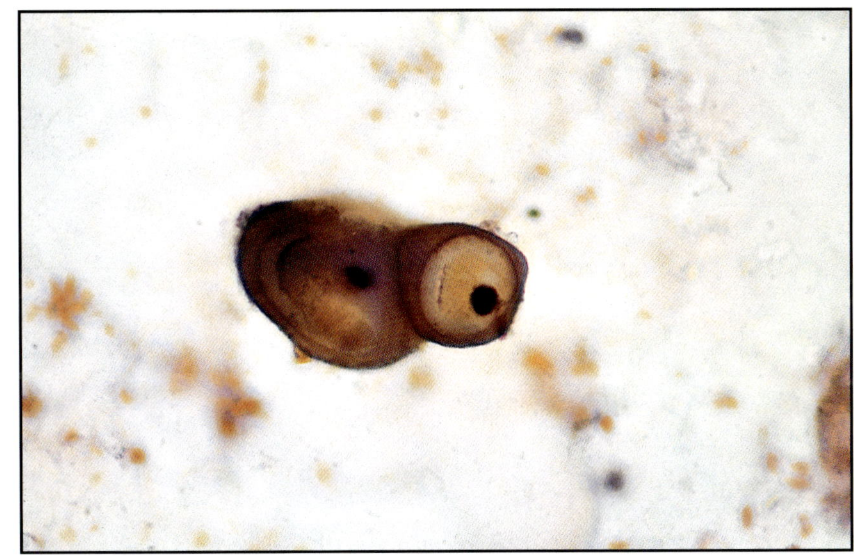

Image 6.29
Heterologous mixed müllerian tumor
of the uterus. A fragment of cartilage
contains numerous atypical chondrocytes and relatively scant cartilaginous
matrix (see Image 6.25). Endometrial
brushing (Papanicolaou, 200X).

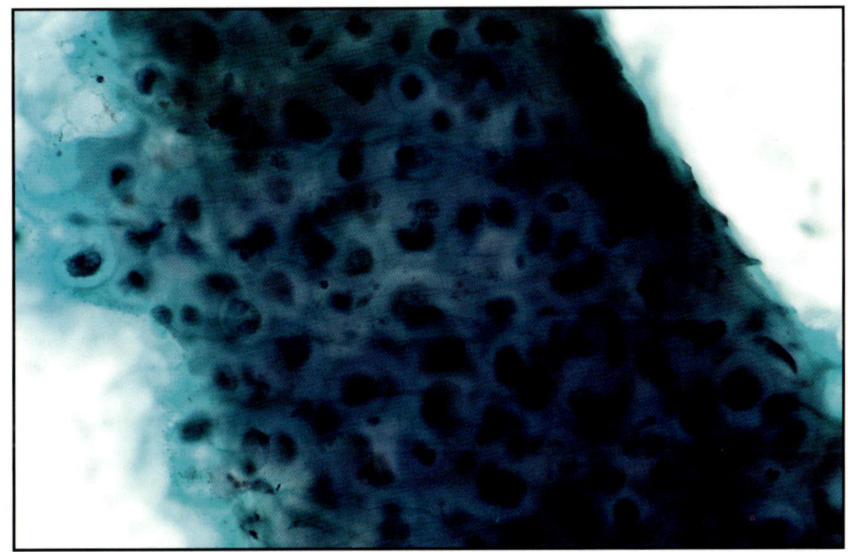

Image 6.30
Heterologous mixed müllerian tumor
of the uterus. Several highly atypical
chondrocytes have pleomorphic, hyperchromatic nuclei and are surrounded by
a ring of cartilaginous matrix. They are
consistent with chondrosarcoma (see
Image 6.25). Endometrial brushing
(Papanicolaou, 400X).

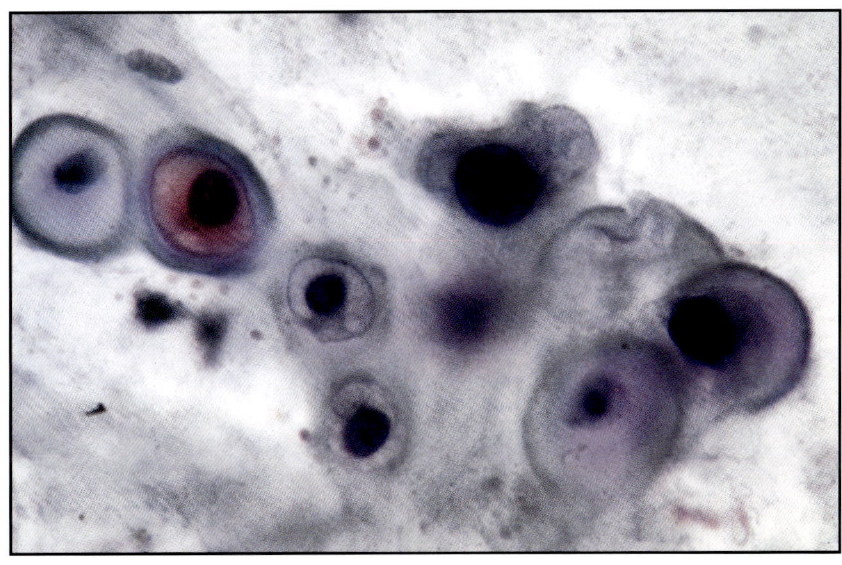

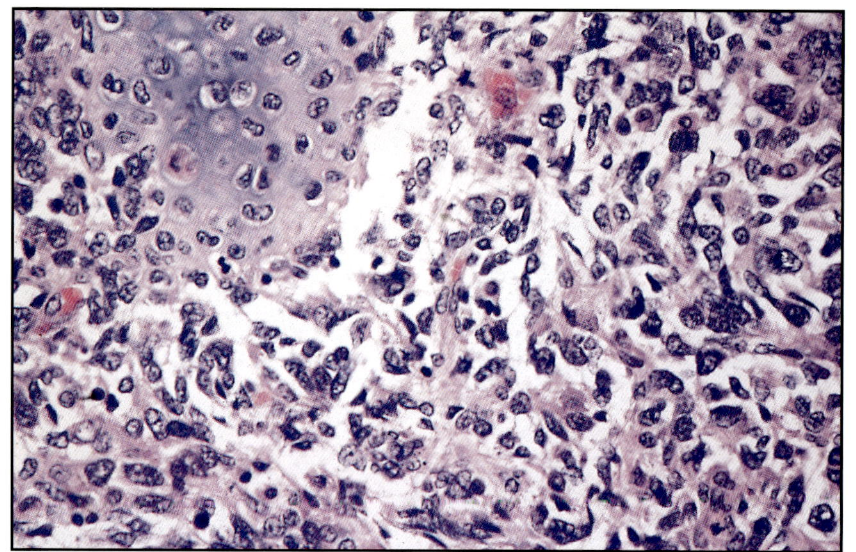

Image 6.31

Heterologous mixed müllerian tumor of the uterus. The tumor is associated with areas of high–grade stromal sarcoma (see Image 6.25), skeletal muscle (not shown in this picture; see Image 6.26), and chondrocytes at different levels of maturation (see Images 6.27-6.30). Histologic section (H&E, 200X).

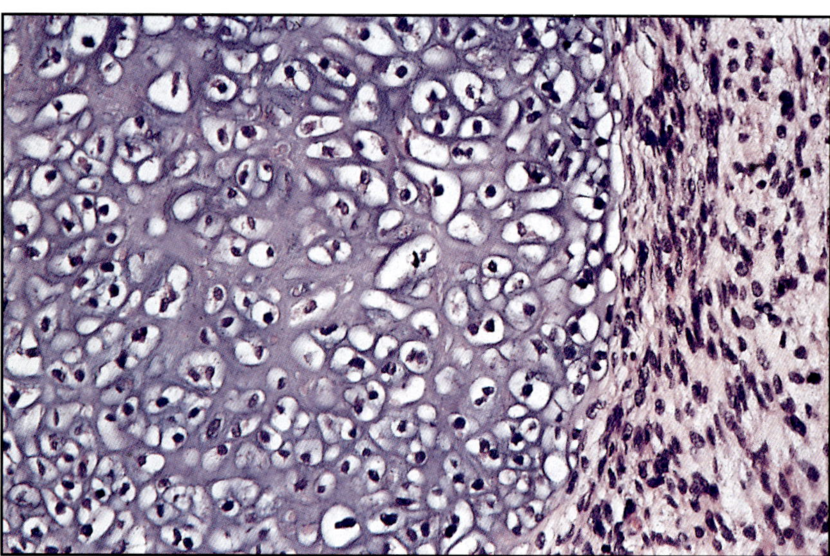

Image 6.32

Heterologous mixed müllerian tumor of the uterus. In one area of the same tumor shown in Image 6.31, cartilaginous differentiation is present. Numerous atypical chondrocytes, some of which are binucleated (see Images 6.29 and 6.30), are consistent with chondrosarcoma. Histologic section (H&E, 200X).

References

1. Aaro LA, Symmonds RE, Dockerty MB: Sarcoma of the uterus: A clinical and pathologic study of 177 cases. *Am J Obstet Gynecol* 94: 101–109, 1966.

2. Enzinger FM, Weiss SW: *Soft Tissue Tumors.* St Louis, MO, CV Mosby Co, 1983, pp 298–324.

3. Fekete PS, Vellios F: The clinical and histologic spectrum of endometrial stromal neoplasms: A report of 41 cases. *Int J Gynecol Pathol* 3:198, 1984.

4. Hendrickson MR, Kempson RL: *Surgical Pathology of the Uterine Corpus.* Philadelphia, PA, WB Saunders Co, 1980.

5. Kempson RL, Bari W: Uterine sarcoma: Classification, diagnosis, and prognosis. *Hum Pathol* 1:331–349, 1970.

6 Oda Y, Nakanishi I, Tateiwa T: Intramural müllerian adenosarcoma of the uterus with adenomyosis. *Arch Pathol Lab Med* 108:798–801, 1984.

7. Rosai J: *Ackerman's Surgical Pathology.* 7th ed. St Louis, MO, CV Mosby Co, 1989, pp 1050–1097.

8. Silverberg SG: Reproducibility of the mitosis count in the histologic diagnosis of smooth muscle tumors of the uterus. *Hum Pathol* 7:451–454, 1976.

9. Tao LC, Davidson DD: Aspiration biopsy cytology of smooth muscle tumors: A cytologic approach to the differentiation between leiomyosarcoma and leiomyoma. *Acta Cytol* 37:300–308, 1993.

10. Wile AG, Evans HL, Romsdahl MM: Leiomyosarcoma of the soft tissue: A clinicopathologic study. *Cancer* 48:1022–1032, 1981.

11. Zaloudek CJ, Norris HJ: Mesenchymal tumors of the uterus. In: *Progress in Surgical Pathology, III,* Fenoglio CM, Wolff M (editors). New York, NY, Masson Publishing Inc, 1981, pp 1–35.

◙ Index

Numbers in **boldface** refer to pages on which images, tables, and figures appear.